Action Research
in Healthcare

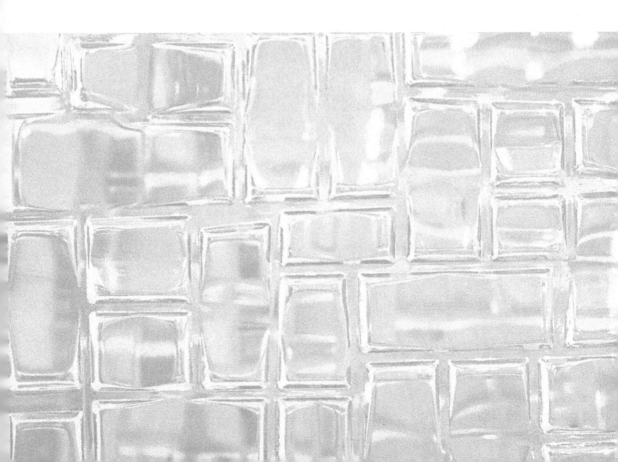

Action Research
in Healthcare

**Elizabeth Koshy,
Valsa Koshy and
Heather Waterman**

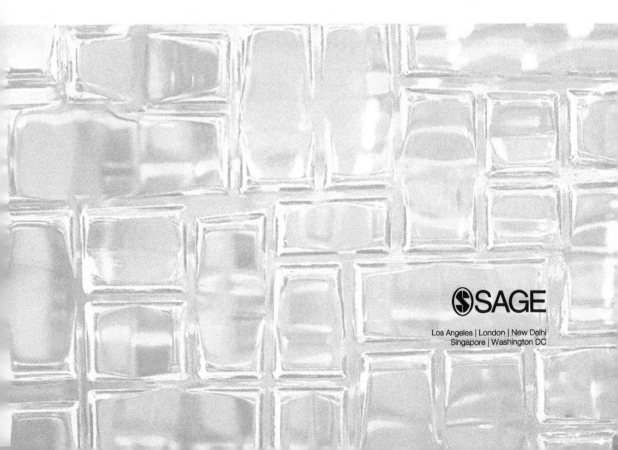

◆SAGE

Los Angeles | London | New Delhi
Singapore | Washington DC

First published 2011

SAGE Publications Ltd
1 Oliver's Yard
55 City Road
London EC1Y 1SP

SAGE Publications Inc.
2455 Teller Road
Thousand Oaks, California 91320

SAGE Publications India Pvt Ltd
B 1/I 1 Mohan Cooperative Industrial Area
Mathura Road
New Delhi 110 044

SAGE Publications Asia-Pacific Pte Ltd
33 Pekin Street #02-01
Far East Square
Singapore 048763

Library of Congress Control Number: 2010926689

British Library Cataloguing in Publication data

A catalogue record for this book is available from the British Library.

ISBN 978-1-84860-188-8
ISBN 978-1-84860-189-5 (pbk)

Typeset by C&M Digitals (P) Ltd, Chennai, India

Contents

About the authors

Dr Elizabeth Koshy is a General Practitioner who works as a Clinical Research Fellow at Imperial College, London. She studied the use of a range of research methodologies during her studies for a Master's in Epidemiology at the London School of Hygiene and Tropical Medicine (University of London); since then she has been carrying out research whilst on fellowship from the National Institute for Health Research (NIHR). She is currently funded by a doctoral fellowship from the NIHR. In her varied roles, she has realized the potential of the action research approach in the context of healthcare, especially within general practice. Dr Koshy also brings in her experience of working in hospitals, Primary Care settings, and as a former tutor for undergraduate medical students at Imperial College, London. All these roles have given her useful insights into the valuable and unique service provided by healthcare workers and how carrying out action research can enhance their professional development and improve the quality of service provided for users.

Professor Valsa Koshy is a Professor of Education and Director of a Research and Development centre at Brunel University. She has led several action research projects commissioned by the UK Department of Education and other public bodies. She continues to support practising teachers and advisers in several Local Authorities to undertake action research projects. She teaches on the Master's and Doctoral programmes at the university and supervizes doctoral students. She brings her expertise in training, teaching and evaluating practices into this book. She has a strong interest in participatory research, which she believes empowers practitioners. Professor Koshy has written several books and articles. Her book *Action Research for Improving Educational Practice*, also published by SAGE, is often described by readers as *very accessible* and *practical*.

Professor Heather Waterman is Professor of Nursing and Ophthalmology at Manchester University. She leads an ophthalmology nursing research team with a special interest in adherence and glaucoma. She has a long-standing interest in participatory research methodologies and has contributed to the development of action research in healthcare in many different roles: as an academic supporting action researchers, as a prolific writer of journal articles on the use of action research in healthcare settings and as an authoritative member of several bodies which review action research proposals and academic papers. She has led a systematic review and guidance for assessment of action research (Waterman et al., 2001) which is widely quoted in almost all publications relating to action research in healthcare settings. Her research portfolio consists of numerous academic and professional publications and she has been either lead or collaborator on externally funded grants from charities, industry, the Department of Health in the UK and the National Institute for Health Research, UK.

Acknowledgements

We are indebted to many people and organizations for supporting us in writing this book, which is designed to assist healthcare workers when carrying out action research. Although it is impossible for us to list all the people who have influenced our thinking and experiences over the years, we would like to express our gratitude to all of them. We would wish to send our special thanks to the following:

- Our colleagues and students who have worked with us on action research projects. We have learnt a great deal from our students, both at undergraduate and post-graduate levels, and have seen first hand the level of enthusiasm, excitement, and commitment of these people which has convinced us of the unique opportunities provided by action research for improving practice.
- We would thank all the students who have given us permission to use extracts from their work and quote their experiences in this book.
- We would wish to acknowledge the help given by Catrin Pinheiro-Torres who assisted us with our literature search and with the chapter on data analysis.
- Our gratitude also goes to Alison Poyner, at SAGE, for her guidance and for understanding the unexpected pressures the authors faced during the writing of this book.
- This book is dedicated to Elizabeth's daughter and Valsa's granddaughter Colette and to Heather's mother Jo.

Introduction

Action research is increasingly being used as a research approach across disciplines in healthcare, social work, and education. This book has been written as a practical guide for health workers who are interested in finding out what action research means and what it entails, either because they are involved in or intend to be involved in action research projects. Those who may be planning to lead action research projects should also find the book useful. In the world we live in – with its increased accountability and financial restrictions – providing the best possible healthcare, which is the ultimate goal shared by all those who are involved, is a major challenge. We believe that action research provides a methodology which offers an effective way for evaluating and reflecting on what we do, with the aim of improving practice. Carrying out action research involves improving our own learning regardless of whatever role we take in this process, whether it be as facilitators in projects or as members of teams within communities undertaking collaborative projects. The action researcher must constantly ask two all-important questions: What am I doing? How can I improve what I am doing? Carrying out sound action research projects does not happen by accident; it requires systematic working and the continual development of effective strategies.

An important point to make when carrying out action research projects is that these can enhance the professional development of researchers through the learning opportunities these provide. As preparation for writing this book we spoke to a number of health workers and the conversations we had were highly illuminating. Without exception, all of them were inspired at the thought of undertaking research, although some of them also told us that they considered research activities to be largely the sole domain of academics and not really something they were likely to be involved in. When we shared accounts of practitioners' action research projects with one diabetic nurse practitioner (Helen) she had this to say:

> Well, I don't really see myself as a researcher, but listening to you I can see how it would be useful. You see, I do my job, I see diabetic patients and explain to

them the importance of controlling their blood sugar readings and exercise. By being involved in an action research project seeking practical ways of helping them to achieve better control, I can see that both my ability to do what I am doing and the quality of how I deal with the patients could be enhanced. The idea of sharing the research with my colleagues and involving patients in projects really appeals to me.

The perception that research is something undertaken by others 'out there' is common amongst practitioners in other disciplines as well. The following statement from another practitioner, who had been part of an action research project with the second author of this book, reflects how practitioners – irrespective of the professional contexts in which they work – may view the opportunity of being action researchers.

Being involved in action research was gratifying, the experience helped me to consider aspects of my work which needed redirection and rejuvenation. Before that elevating experience, I assumed that all forms of research were the exclusive province of academic researchers in universities. Gaining access to that ivory tower has enabled one practitioner – me – to illuminate sound strategies to work with colleagues in exploring new strategies, implementing ideas, and assessing the effectiveness of the ideas we introduced.

Our own professional experiences have guided and informed the contents of this book. As a General Practitioner, the first author has experienced the power of collaborative work in family practices in improving patient care. Having had extensive training and experience in traditional research methods, her own strong belief is that action research with its practical orientation and collaborative work has much to offer healthcare professionals, whether this is in implementing new initiatives from the government, or making changes to practices in response to new clinical guidance or new research evidence and other developments. She has also grown to understand, first hand, the effectiveness of all professionals working together to implement change. Her personal belief is that there is more potential in the use of the action research approach within general practice. A literature search supports the view that there are far fewer published action research studies in general practice than, say, in nursing and other healthcare settings.

There are abundant examples of action research in educational settings. In fact, many of the references used in books and journal articles relating to action research in healthcare come from education. The contents of this book draw on the personal experiences of the second author, spanning more than fifteen years, in guiding action researchers in various educational settings and working with Master's and doctoral students from various disciplines who were carrying out action research. During that time, she has witnessed the enthusiasm of practitioners in conducting action research, the pride they feel in disseminating their findings, and the level of increased professional confidence they display.

The third author has contributed to the development of action research in healthcare as an action researcher herself in many different roles: as an academic supporting action researchers, as a prolific writer of journal articles on the use of action research in healthcare settings, and as an authoritative member of several bodies which review action research proposals and academic papers. She has led a systematic review and guidance for the assessment of action research (Waterman et al., 2001) which is widely quoted in almost all publications relating to action research in healthcare settings. All three of us have brought our own expertise and experience to bear on this book which we hope will offer support and guidance to our readers.

As the main purpose here is to offer practical guidance to those who intend to carry out action research and those others who are involved in action research projects, we address four important questions:

- What is action research?
- When is it appropriate for practitioners to carry out action research?
- What are the processes involved in conducting action research?
- How can action researchers disseminate their experiences?

We have attempted to address all four of these questions in this book. To begin with, it would be useful to consider the reasons why we may wish to undertake action research. Doing such research facilitates evaluation and personal critical reflection in order to implement necessary changes in practice with greater understanding. Those who are involved in action research construct their own understandings through their practical involvement in the process which is quite different to just reading about various aspects of healthcare. They feel empowered through their active involvement. As new initiatives are introduced with greater frequency within healthcare all over the world, practitioners can often be left with conflicting viewpoints, doubts, and dilemmas which need exploration, evaluation, and reflection. Evaluating and reflecting on one's own practices is an integral part of applied disciplines such as healthcare, social work, and education.

In this book, we hope to address the needs of those who wish to undertake action research as an aspect of their practice. These projects may be facilitated by external funding or may be the outcome of a local necessity to change practice; they may also be a result of an evaluation of the effectiveness of an innovation or a new initiative. In addition action research may be carried out as part of obtaining an educational qualification. Undertaking an action research project involves looking at issues in depth, gathering and assessing the evidence, and then critically reflecting as new ideas are implemented with a view to changing practice. We believe that carrying out action research is all about developing the act of knowing through observation, listening, analysing, questioning, reflecting, and being involved in generating knowledge. The new knowledge and experiences that result can then inform the researchers' future direction.

We have designed this book in such a way that it can provide guidance on all the key aspects involved in carrying out action research. As one single book cannot address every issue in any great depth, we have included a range of references and further reading, directing the reader to suitable sources if they feel they need greater detail in any of the aspects. We have tried to create a book which offers step-by-step guidance for healthcare practitioners serving the needs of a range of the readership: individual researchers, managers, and leaders who facilitate action research groups and tutors and educators in healthcare. We have also tried to introduce an interactive element into the book, inviting readers to join the authors in exploring various aspects of what is involved in conducting action research. We have carried out an extensive search of the literature of books and recent publications and have included examples and case studies, from different contexts in healthcare, in the book.

The information is presented in seven chapters. Chapter 1 explores the concept of action research and considers how it is distinctive from other forms of research. Readers are provided with an overview of how action research has developed over the past few decades, its background, and the key concepts of action research – planning, action, evaluation, refinement, reflection, and theory building. Drawing on expert views, the different perspectives and uses of action research are considered. A range of definitions and established models of action research is provided, which should support action researchers to plan their work and also help them to justify the rationale for the choice of action research as a methodology. Key characteristics of the action research approach are discussed. In addition this chapter also includes a discussion of the theoretical underpinnings of action research in order to support the researcher to articulate his or her positioning in terms of ontological and epistemological assumptions. The chapter concludes with a set of examples of action research projects, carried out by practitioners from a variety of healthcare contexts and dealing with a range of topics, encouraging the reader to consider the features of action research.

Chapters 2 to 6 address the various stages of action research. In Chapter 2, we discuss why researchers will select action research as their approach, along with a discussion of the advantages and perceived limitations of this approach. We address some of the criticisms raised against action research as a methodology and set the scene for the practical aspects of undertaking action research. We then explore the views of experts to consider the role of action research in the professional development of the researcher, the relationship between theory and practice, and the notion of change which constitutes a key element in carrying out action research. We also take a look at the processes involved in conducting action research and invite the reader to consider if and how the processes are embedded within the practical examples provided.

In Chapter 3 we discuss the process of undertaking a literature review for the purpose of the action research topic to be studied. A rationale for undertaking research reviews is provided and guidance on how to gather, organize, analyse, and make use of what is reviewed is presented. The selection and use of electronic sources for a literature search are dealt with in this chapter, along with some practical guidance on how to evaluate the sources of literature that can obtained from the Internet.

Chapter 4 offers practical guidelines to action researchers, whether they are about to start a project or are already involved in a project. Quality issues are discussed. We then explore the contexts which are suitable for action research. Although we believe that the stages of action research are not strictly linear, we also believe these should help researchers to think in terms of planning projects in stages, with a built-in flexibility to refine, make adjustments, and change direction within a given structure. Detailed practical guidance is provided on the various steps in action research, taking the reader through all the stages from identifying a topic, planning an action, reflecting, and evaluating. The process of action planning is discussed in detail and a practical planning sheet is provided. Special consideration is given to the important aspect of 'when things don't go according to plan' and this also looks at how to anticipate any potential problems when you are conducting collaborative research.

In Chapter 5 we try to locate the action research approach as a research methodology and discuss its position within three frequently used paradigms. We discuss the different types of instrumentation for gathering data, using practical examples of data collection from healthcare settings. The advantages and limitations of using different methods are discussed. The need to be systematic in the data-gathering process is emphasized. Ethical considerations are also dealt with.

Chapter 6 focuses on one of the most complex issues in any form of research – the analysis of data. Guidance is provided on how the data may be analysed and presented as themes. The use of computer software packages is also discussed. Examples of healthcare practitioners' accounts of data analysis are provided within this chapter, which concludes with a discussion of using evidence and generating knowledge. In addition issues relating to validating claims to knowledge are addressed.

The type of report written by action researchers will depend on their circumstances. Funded research requires a certain format to be followed, whereas a report in the form of a dissertation or thesis for an accredited course will need to follow a different (and often pre-set) format. Examples of writing reports and the processes involved in writing or disseminating any findings are provided in Chapter 7, along with a discussion of the different ways in which we can disseminate such findings. Guidance on how to publish action research in various forms (newsletters, conference presentations and journal articles) is also provided.

What we have attempted to do in this book is to provide the reader with a clear set of practical guidelines for undertaking action research. The examples of action research, in the various healthcare settings, provided within the text, bear testimony to its potential to improve the quality of care for the users as well as helping with the enlightenment and learning processes of those who work within it.

1

What is Action Research?

This chapter focuses on:

- What action research is
- The purposes of conducting action research
- The development of action research
- What is involved in action research
- The models and definitions of action research
- The key characteristics of action research
- The philosophical worldview of the action researcher
- Examples of action research projects.

Introduction

Action research – which is also known as Participatory Action Research (PAR), community-based study, co-operative enquiry, action science and action learning – is an approach commonly used for improving conditions and practices in a range healthcare environments (Lingard et al., 2008; Whitehead et al., 2003). It involves healthcare practitioners conducting systematic enquiries in order to help them improve their own practices, which in turn can enhance their working environment and the working environments of those who are part of it – clients, patients, and users. The purpose of undertaking action research is to bring about change in specific contexts, as Parkin (2009) describes it. Through their observations and communications with other people, healthcare workers are continually making informal evaluations and judgements about what it is they do. The difference between this and carrying out an action research project is that during the process researchers will need to develop and use a range of skills to achieve their aims, such as careful planning, sharpened observation and listening, evaluation, and critical reflection.

Meyer (2000) maintains that action research's strength lies in its focus on generating solutions to practical problems and its ability to empower practitioners, by getting them to engage with research and the subsequent development or implementation activities. Meyer states that practitioners can choose to research their own practice or an outside researcher can be engaged to help to identify any problems, seek and implement practical solutions, and systematically monitor and reflect on the process and outcomes of change. Whitehead et al. (2003) point out that the place of action research in health promotion programmes is an important and yet relatively unacknowledged and understated activity and suggest that this state of affairs denies many health promotion researchers a valuable resource for managing effective changes in practice.

Most of the reported action research studies in healthcare will have been carried out in collaborative teams. The community of enquiry may have consisted of members within a general practice or hospital ward, general practitioners working with medical school tutors, or members within a healthcare clinic. The users of healthcare services can often be included in an action research study; as such they are not *researched on* as is the case in much of traditional research. This may also involve several healthcare practitioners working together within a geographical area. Multidisciplinary teams can often be involved (for example, medical workers working with social work teams). Action research projects may also be initiated and carried out by members of one or two institutions and quite often an external facilitator (from a local university, for example) may be included. All the participating researchers will ideally have to be involved in the process of data collection, data analysis, planning and implementing action, and validating evidence and critical reflection, before applying the findings to improve their own practice or the effectiveness of the system within which they work.

Purposes of conducting action research

In the context of this book, we can say that action research supports practitioners in seeking out ways in which they can provide an enhanced quality of healthcare. With this purpose in mind, the following features of the action research approach are worthy of consideration (Koshy, 2010: 1):

- Action research is a method used for improving practice. It involves action, evaluation, and critical reflection and – based on the evidence gathered – changes in practice are then implemented.

- Action research is participative and collaborative; it is undertaken by individuals with a common purpose.
- It is situation-based and context specific.
- It develops reflection based on interpretations made by the participants.
- Knowledge is created through action and at the point of application.
- Action research can involve problem solving, if the solution to the problem leads to the improvement of practice.
- In action research findings will emerge as action develops, but these are not conclusive or absolute.

Later in this chapter we shall explore the various definitions of action research.

Hughes (2008) presents a convincing argument for carrying out action research in healthcare settings. Quoting the declaration of the World Health Organization (1946) that 'health is a state of complete physical, mental and social well being and not merely the absence of disease or infirmity', Hughes stresses that our health as individuals and communities depends on environmental factors, the quality of our relationships, and our beliefs and attitudes as well as bio-medical factors, and therefore in order to understand our health we must see ourselves as inter-dependent with human and non-human elements in the system we participate in. Hughes adds that the holistic way of understanding health, by looking at the whole person in context, is congruent with the participative paradigm of action research. The following extract coming from an action researcher (included by Reason and Bradbury in the introduction to their *Handbook of Action Research*) sums up the key notion of action research being a useful approach for healthcare professionals:

> For me it is really a quest for life, to understand life and to create what I call living knowledge – knowledge which is valid for the people with whom I work and for myself. (Marja Liisa Swantz, in Reason and Bradbury, 2001: 1)

So what is this living knowledge? As Reason and Bradbury (2001: 2) explain, the primary purpose of action research is to produce practical knowledge that is useful to people in the everyday conduct of their lives. They maintain that action research is about working towards practical outcomes and that it is also about 'creating new forms of understanding, since action without reflection and understanding is blind, just as theory without action is meaningless' and that the participatory nature of action research 'makes it only possible *with*, *for* and *by* persons and communities, ideally involving all stakeholders both in the questioning and sense making that informs the research, and in the action which is its focus'. Meyer (2000) describes action research as a process that involves people and social situations that have the ultimate aim of changing an existing situation for the better.

In the following sections of this chapter we will trace the development of action research as a methodology over the past few decades and then consider the different perspectives and models provided by experts in the field. Different models and definitions of action research are explored and an attempt is made to identify the unique features of action research that should make it an attractive mode of research for healthcare practitioners. Examples of action research projects undertaken by healthcare practitioners in a range of situations are provided later in this chapter.

The development of action research: a brief background

Whether the reader is a novice or is progressing with an action research project, it would be useful to be aware of how action research has developed as a method for carrying out research over the past few decades. The work of Kurt Lewin (1946), who researched extensively on social issues, is often described as a major landmark in the development of action research as a methodology. Lewin's work was followed by that of Stephen Corey and others in the USA, who applied this methodology for researching into educational issues. In Britain, according to Hopkins (2002), the origins of action research can be traced back to the Schools Council's Humanities Curriculum Project (1967–72) with its emphasis on an experimental curriculum and the re-conceptualisation of curriculum development. The most well known proponent of action research in the UK has been Lawrence Stenhouse, whose seminal (1975) work *An Introduction to Curriculum Research and Development* added to the appeal of action research for studying the theory and practice of teaching and the curriculum. In turn, educational action researchers including Elliott (1991) have influenced action researchers in healthcare settings.

What is involved in action research?

Research is about generating knowledge. Action research creates knowledge based on enquiries conducted within specific and often practical contexts. As articulated earlier, the purpose of action research is to learn through action that then leads on to personal or professional development. Action research is participatory in nature, which led

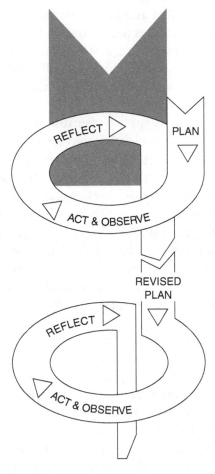

FIGURE 1.1 *Kemmis and McTaggart's action research spiral*

Kemmis and McTaggart (2000: 595) to describe it as *participatory research*. The authors state that action research involves a spiral of self-reflective cycles of:

- Planning a change.
- Acting and observing the process and consequences of the change.
- Reflecting on these processes and consequences and then replanning.
- Acting and observing.
- Reflecting.
- And so on ...

Figure 1.1 illustrates the spiral model of action research proposed by Kemmis and McTaggart (2000: 564), although the authors do not recommend that this is used as a rigid structure. They maintain that in reality the process may not be as neat as the spiral of self-contained cycles of planning, acting and observing, and reflecting suggests. These stages, they maintain, will *overlap*, and initial plans will quickly become obsolete in the light of learning from experience. In reality the process is likely to be more fluid, open, and responsive.

We find the spiral model appealing because it gives an opportunity to visit a phenomenon at a higher level each time and so to progress towards a greater overall understanding. By carrying out action research using this model, one can understand a particular issue within a healthcare context and make informed decisions with an enhanced understanding. It is therefore about empowerment. However, Winter and Munn-Giddings (2001) point out that the spiral model may suggest that even the basic process may take a long time to complete. A review of examples of studies included in this book and the systematic review of studies using the action research approach by Waterman et al. (2001) show that the period of a project has varied significantly, ranging from a few months to one or two years.

Several other models have also been put forward by those who have studied different aspects of action research and we shall present some of these later in this section. Our purpose in doing so is to enable the reader to analyse the principles involved in these models which should, in turn, lead to a deeper understanding of the processes involved in action research. No specific model is being recommended here and as the reader may have already noticed they have many similarities. Action researchers should always adopt the models which suit their purpose best or adapt these for use.

The model employed by Elliot (1991: 71) shares many of the features of that of Kemmis and McTaggart and is based on Lewin's work of the 1940s. It includes identifying a general idea, reconnaissance or fact-finding, planning, action, evaluation, amending plan and taking second action step, and so on, as can be seen in Figure 1.2. Other models, such as O'Leary's (2004: 141) cycles of action research shown in Figure 1.3, portray action research as a cyclic process which takes shape as knowledge emerges.

In O'Leary's model, for example, it is stressed that 'cycles converge towards better situation understanding and improved action implementation; and are based in evaluative practice that alters between action and critical reflection' (2004: 140). O'Leary sees action research as an experiential learning approach, to change, where the goal is to continually refine the methods, data, and interpretation in light of the understanding developed in each earlier cycle.

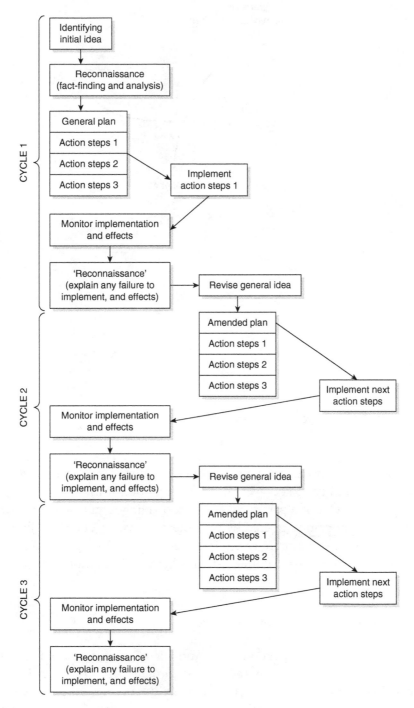

FIGURE 1.2 *Elliot's action research model.*

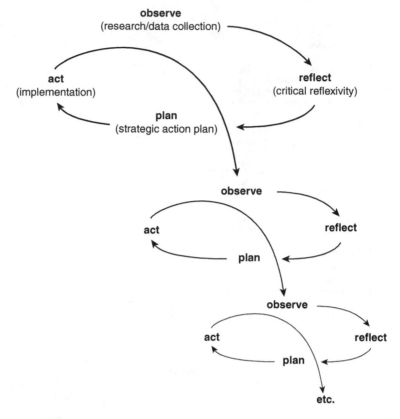

FIGURE 1.3   *O'Leary's cycles of research*

Although it is useful to consider different models, we must include a word of caution here. Excessive reliance on a particular model, or following the stages or cycles of a particular model too rigidly, could adversely affect the unique opportunity offered by the emerging nature and flexibility that are the hallmarks of action research. The models of practice presented in this chapter are not intended to offer a straitjacket to fit an enquiry.

Definitions of action research

Closely related to the purposes and models of action research are the various definitions of action research. Although there is no universally accepted definition for action research, many useful ones do exist. We shall consider some of these in this section. Reason and Bradbury (2006) describe action research as an approach which is used in designing studies which seek both to inform and influence practice. The authors state that action research is a particular orientation and purpose of enquiry rather than a research methodology. They also propose that action research consists of a 'family of approaches' that have different orientations, yet reflect the characteristics which seek to 'involve, empower and improve' aspects of participants' social world. A further list of features of action research, put forward by the same authors (2008: 3), states that it:

- is a set of practices that respond to people's desire to act creatively in the face of practical and often pressing issues in their lives in organizations and communities;
- calls for an engagement with people in collaborative relationships, opening new 'communicative spaces' in which dialogue and development can flourish;
- draws on many ways of knowing, both in the evidence that is generated in inquiry and its expression in diverse forms of presentation as we share our learning with wider audiences;
- is value oriented, seeking to address issues of significance concerning the flourishing of human persons, their communities, and the wider ecology in which we participate;
- is a living, emergent process that cannot be pre-determined but changes and develops as those engaged deepen their understanding of the issues to be addressed and develop their capacity as co-inquirers both individually and collectively.

At this point, it may be useful to explore some of the other definitions and observations on action research as a methodology offered by various authors. We define action research as an approach employed by practitioners for improving practice as part of the process of change. The research is context-bound and participative. It is a continuous learning process in which the researcher learns and also shares the newly generated knowledge with those who may benefit from it. In the context of practitioner research, Hopkins (2002) maintains that action research combines a substantive act with a research procedure and that it is action disciplined by enquiry and a personal attempt at understanding, while engaged in a process of improvement and reform. Cohen and Manion describe the emergent nature of action research in their definition and maintain that action research is:

> essentially an on-the-spot procedure designed to deal with a concrete problem located in an immediate situation. This means that ideally, the step-by-step process is constantly monitored over varying periods of time and by a variety of mechanisms (questionnaires, diaries, interviews and case studies, for example) so that the ensuing feedback may be translated into modifications, adjustment, directional changes, redefinitions, as necessary, so as to bring about lasting benefit to the ongoing process itself rather than to some future occasion (1994: 192).

In their systematic review of action research, Waterman et al. (2001: 4) provide a comprehensive and practically useful definition:

> Action research is a period of inquiry, which describes, interprets and explains social situations while executing a change of intervention aimed at improvement and involvement. It is problem-focused, context specific and future-orientated. Action research is a group activity with an explicit value basis and is founded on a partnership between action researchers and participants, all of whom are involved in the change process. The participatory process is educative and empowering, involving a dynamic approach in which problem-identification, planning, action and evaluation are interlinked. Knowledge may be advanced through reflection and research, and qualitative and quantitative research methods may be employed to collect data. Different types of knowledge may be produced by action research, including practical and propositional. Theory may be generated and refined and its general application explored through cycles of the action research process.

Finally, Winter and Munn-Giddings's (2001: 8) definition of action research, as a 'study of a social situation carried out by those involved in that situation in order to improve both their practice and the quality of their understanding', captures the essence of the philosophy underlying the action research approach.

A careful study of the definitions and viewpoints we have presented in this section should help to highlight some of the unique features of action research. The key concepts include *a better understanding, participation, improvement, reform, problem finding, problem solving, a step-by-step process, modification,* and *theory building*. These words also perhaps demonstrate the reasons for the popularity of action research as a mode of study for healthcare professionals.

Key characteristics of action research

Many attempts have been made, over the years, to identify the characteristics that highlight the uniqueness of action research and distinguish it from other methodologies. Carr and Kemmis (1986: 164) in their seminal text on action research included the underlying principles of the action research approach. These include its

- participatory character;
- democratic impulse;
- simultaneous contribution to social science (knowledge) and social change (practice).

In the *British Medical Journal*, Meyer (2000) explains these three characteristics from a practical perspective which is presented in detail in the following section as this has some important information and practical guidance for action researchers.

Meyer contends that *participation* is fundamental in action research as it is an approach which demands that participants perceive the need to change and are willing to play an active part in the research and change process. Conflicts may arise in the course of the research. It is vital that outside researchers working with practitioners must obtain their trust and agree the rules for the control of the data and their use, as well as acknowledging how any potential conflict will be resolved.

In order to address the feature of *democratic impulse*, according to Meyer, this requires participants to be seen as equals. The researcher works as a facilitator of change, consulting with participants not only on the action process but also on how it will be evaluated. One benefit to this is that it can make the research process and outcomes more meaningful to practitioners by rooting these in the reality of day-to-day practice. Throughout the research process the findings are fed back to participants for validation. In the formative process involved in the spirals of planning, observing, reflecting, and re-planning care needs to be taken because this can be threatening, something which is common in healthcare settings.

With regard to the role of action research to contribute to social science and social change, Meyer highlights the concern about the theory-practice gap in clinical practice; practitioners have to rely on their intuition and experience since traditional scientific knowledge – for example, the results of randomized controlled trials – often do not seem to fit with the uniqueness of the situation. Action research, Meyer maintains, is one way of dealing with this because it draws on a practitioner's situation and experience and can therefore generate findings that are meaningful to them. In this context we are thus made aware of an important feature – that the contributions to knowledge arising from action research and any generalizations are different from other conventional forms of research. Reports from action research projects will rely on readers underwriting the accounts by drawing on their own knowledge of human situations and therefore it is important for action researchers to describe their work in rich contextual detail.

Philosophical worldview of an action researcher

Research is a form of disciplined enquiry leading to the generation of knowledge. The knowledge your research generates is derived from a range of approaches. Your approach to research may vary according to the context of your study, your beliefs, the strategies you employ, and the methods you use. The research paradigm (a collection of assumptions and beliefs which will guide you along the path to conducting research and interpreting findings) you select will be guided both by your subject discipline and your beliefs. Action research is a specific method of conducting research by health professionals with the ultimate aim of improving practice. Your epistemological and ontological views may influence your research and the research methods you use.

When conducting research of any kind, a consideration of the philosophical stance or worldview (Guba and Lincoln, 1990) is important. Creswell (2009: 6) describes a worldview as a 'general orientation about the world and the nature of the research that the researcher holds'. In an attempt to position action research within a research paradigm we think it may be useful to discuss the positivist, interpretivist, and participatory worldviews here. The positivist paradigm is based on a belief in an objective reality which can be gained from observable data. This worldview is often referred to as scientific method and the knowledge gained is based on careful observation and measuring the objective reality that exists 'out there' (Creswell, 2009). This method relies on quantitative measures and the relationships between variables are highlighted.

Interpretivism, which has emerged as a worldview developed in the social sciences, allows for a departure from positivist constraints. Qualitative methods such as phenomenology, ethnography, grounded theory, and narrative research are used within this paradigm which is based on the belief that knowledge is socially constructed, subjective, and influenced by culture and social interactions. Within this worldview, the researcher gathers data while still retaining their objectivity.

Waterman et al. (2001) provide an illuminating account of the philosophical perspectives that underpin action research in healthcare. They highlight that the most influential of these is *critical theory*, which draws on the writings of Jürgen Habermas (1971, 1984). Waterman et al. also state that this approach arose from a desire to democratize research in order to present a challenge to the institutionalization of research which was viewed as being exclusive and exploitative. One aim here is to encourage those who are actually excluded from the process of informing it, thereby making it participatory. Linked to this is a desire for social improvement: the Aristotelian notion of praxis – of acting on the conditions of one's situation in order to change them (Meyer, 1995) – and Kemmis and McTaggart's (2000) argument that to study practice means to change it, but also, that practice is changed in order to study it. Waterman et al. (2001) maintain that in this approach value is attached to both qualitative and quantitative research methods; these are seen as complementary. However, critics of this approach would argue that it is idealistic and the desire to create a more just healthcare system is both naive and optimistic.

Some experts would hold the view that action research is located in the *participatory worldview* and that it is unique because it is context-bound and involves action which is designed to change local situations. The researcher is involved in the research process which informs practice and knowledge is generated from practice. As Punch (2009: 135) describes it, 'the central idea is conveyed by the term action research'. Action researchers 'engage in careful diligent enquiry not for the purpose of discovering new facts or revising accepted laws or theories, but to acquire information having practical application to the solution of specific problems related to their work' (Stringer, 2004: 3).

Theoretical positioning of the action researcher

The essence of the type of enquiry conducted by an action researcher is that it involves an investigation of some component or aspect of a social system. Such a system is composed of humans engaged in interaction, using gestures and language, resulting in the creation of impressions and the transmission of information. The quest for knowledge – to be conveyed as information – has its historical roots in metaphysics, which may be regarded as a quest for some form of immutable reality that exists behind the face of changing, transient, social entities. The physical sciences inherited this quest and established forms for the various fundamental, atomic components of our world. The social sciences in embracing action research are driven by the pursuit of meanings and interpretations which are socially constructed, thus forming the systems of belief and understanding that direct and enrich the lives of human beings.

For social systems some would argue that a postmodernist approach looks for knowledge within a social system, as opposed to the positivist approach which demands logical or scientific support for beliefs. They hold the view that action research does not subscribe to a positivist viewpoint concerning evidence and the conclusions inherent in a research exercise and would argue for a postmodernist attitude to epistemology (theory of knowledge) – advocating questions and discussions within the research exercise – so that emerging beliefs, whilst not embedded in an immutable reality, are the product of a negotiated consensus that contributes to a future harmony of actions and elevations of the life course. The authors of this book would leave the reader to position themself within a view which they feel is compatible with their beliefs and convictions.

Making the researcher's philosophical stance known

When selecting and making a decision about what methodology to use, and to adopt while also reporting on findings, researchers will need to consider their ontological and epistemological stance. Whichever philosophical stance they take, it is important to declare this and understand the implications of doing so with regard to data collection and analysis. In order to do that we need to take closer look, in the next section, at what the different theoretical perspectives mean within the context of action research.

Ontological issues

The term 'ontology' is used to designate the theory of being. Its mandate is the development of strategies which can illuminate the components of people's *social reality* – about what exists, what it looks like, the units that make it up, and how these units interact with each other (Blaikie, 1993: 6). Within action research, researchers would consider this reality as socially constructed and not external and independent. The meaningful construction occurs through interpretations of researchers' experiences and communication. The stories they tell will be based on subjective accounts from the people who live within their environment. The methods of data collection they use will be consistent with their ontological stance. Action researchers must ideally make their theoretical stance clear at the start and also at the dissemination stage.

Epistemological issues

The term 'epistemology' is used to designate the theory of knowledge and it presents a view and justification for what can be regarded as knowledge – what can be known and the criteria that knowledge must satisfy in order to be called knowledge rather than beliefs (Blaikie, 1993: 7). For traditional researchers, knowledge is certain and can be discovered through scientific means. For an action researcher, the nature of knowledge and what constitutes knowledge are different. The type of data collected is more subjective where the experience and insights are of a unique and personal nature (Burrell and Morgan, 1979). What people say and how we interpret what they do and say are important for an action researcher for knowledge creation. Again, in any reporting of their research and claims to knowledge generation, action researchers need to acknowledge their epistemological stance.

Further reading is also provided at the end of the chapter for those who wish to delve deeper into these issues.

Some practical examples of action research projects

In the following section, four examples of published action research projects will be presented. These projects, set within different contexts and locations, are included here for the explicit purpose of introducing readers to what has been reported previously as action research studies. These are presented here as summaries, while keeping them as close as possible to the original published papers in order to capture the contexts and situations in which they were located, as well as to attempt to present the viewpoints of the researchers in their own words. (We would, however, recommend reading the full version of each paper; full references for all these can be found in the reference section.) And while you may as yet be unfamiliar with the technical terminology used in the papers, these accounts should introduce you to the key concepts involved in action research.

Each project is presented in the same format; it starts with the background of the study, which is followed by the methods used, and then presents any outcomes. Each example concludes with the researchers' commentary on why they selected action research as their research approach.

While reading these examples, based on what has been reported by the researchers themselves, it would be useful to consider *whether and how* their experiences relate to the different models and definitions presented earlier in this chapter. These published examples (where researchers have stated that they have used an action research approach) are presented for the purpose of encouraging critical reflection; we hope the reader will examine each one critically and make an initial appraisal of whether and in what way they reflect the principles and features of action research.

Example 1.1   Development of an information source for patients and the public about general practice services: an action research study (Marshall et al., 2006)

Background

Publishing of information about the performance of healthcare providers is regarded as central to promoting greater accountability and empowering patients to exercise choice. Marshall et al. state that the aim of the study was to explore the information needs of patients in the context of UK Primary Care and to develop an information source about general practice services that was designed to be usable and useful to patients. This project was set against the background of a national call that highlighted a need to provide better and more accessible information about the performance of health-care providers, something that was considered essential if the health services were to become more orientated around the needs of patients and members of the public.

Methods

The study was conducted using an action research approach, making use of data gathering from formal and informal interviews, focus groups, participant observation, and a review of documents. The setting was the geographical areas covered by two Primary Care Trusts in the North of England and two Local Health Boards in South Wales. The participants included 103 members of the public, general practice staff from 19 practices, National Health Service (NHS) managers from four Primary Care organizations, and the research team.

   The Primary Care Organizations (PCOs) were selected on the basis of their geographical proximity to the research bases, their willingness to participate in the projects, and their contrasting demographic and organizational character-istics. The research team worked with a senior member of the management team who 'championed' the project and recruited up to six volunteer practices. Each of the practices agreed to work with their patients, PCO managers, and the research team to develop and publish information about their services and performance. Patient participators were drawn from established practice-based patient participation groups, or from individuals who had responded to advertisements in the various practice waiting rooms. While these were volun-teers they included representatives from both genders, all social classes, and adults from all age groups.

   Data were collected using a multi-method process, which emphasized the iterations between defining the issues, developing solutions, and evaluating. In-depth interviews were carried out with PCO members, managers, and practice staff. Data were also gathered via focus group meetings (conducted with patients registered with the practice and with practice staff), informal meetings with practice staff and PCO managers, and by participant observation of PCOs. Practice meetings (including patient participation/support groups meetings), backed up by fieldnotes, research dairies, and a review of relevant documentation – such as annual reports and minutes of meetings – also provided datasets.

Data (field notes, interview transcripts, reflective diaries, and documents) were analysed using a *constant comparative* approach. The research team identified emerging themes from participants' discussions that described the factors influencing the public's use of information and their information needs. Themes were explored and interpreted in an interactive way with the project participants and were then triangulated between the different stakeholder groups and sites. The findings were used in turn to guide the development of an information source for patients and the public about general practice services.

Overview of outcomes

The research team found that the public wanted to know more about the quality and range of general practice services, but the sources of information then current did not meet their needs. The public did not like league tables that compared the performance of various practices and only a small number of people wanted to use comparative information to choose between practices. They seemed to be more interested in the content and availability of services and the willingness of practices to improve than in each practice's absolute relative performance. They also wanted to be clear about the source of the information in order to be able to make personal judgements about its veracity. Information was most likely to be useful if it adhered to the basic principle of cognitive science in terms of its structure, content, and presentation format. Using these findings, paper and electronic prototype versions of a guide to general practice services were developed.

Researchers' comments on the use of the action research approach

The authors chose action research as an approach because it was felt to be compatible with the participation and developmental nature of the project and with their desire to empower service users and generate a tangible product. The nature of the complex processes and the role of the researchers as facilitators of change was felt to be compatible with an action research approach. The action research approach also enabled the research team to act as partners in the process, with all of the participants sharing views and contributing to the change processes, according to their knowledge and expertise.

Example 1.2   Valuing autonomy, struggling for an identity and a collective voice, and seeking role recognition: community mental health nurses' perception of their roles (White and Kudless, 2008)

Background

This study was carried out in a large, community-based, behavioural health system that was located in the south east United States and offered a wide range of programmes to provide a full continuum of care, including mental health, substance abuse, and mental retardation services. Programmes such as a Detoxification Unit, PACT (Programs for Assertive Community Treatment) Teams, and Group Homes employed 40 Community Mental Health Nurses (CMHNs). These CMHNs were educated to all levels and assumed different jobs. Nurses, with basic level education work on PACT teams utilizing a case management approach, managed medication clinics or worked as staff nurses in the Detoxification Unit. Those with a Master's qualification worked as Clinical Nurse Specialists or Nurse Practitioners. Clinical Nurse Specialists (called Senior Clinicians) worked alongside other senior clinicians, such as social workers and psychologists or interdisciplinary teams, providing intake evaluations, treatment, and consultations. In this system Nurse Practitioners functioned primarily as psychopharmacology prescribers and treated the complex co-morbid conditions of the consumers. Nurses felt they were 'chained to clerical work' and this left them frustrated at not being able to use their nursing skills directly on behalf of consumers. They expressed their frustration resulting from this situation.

Leaders of this community mental health system approached the problem of job frustration, moral issues, and the turnover concerns of their Community Mental Health Nurses (CMHNs) by designing a study using Participatory Action Research Methodology (PAR). The goal was to understand and resolve CMHNs' frustrations. A consultant researcher was hired to assist the nurses with outlining their concerns and problems and worked with them in giving 'voice' to their frustrations.

Methods

Critical theory was 'both a philosophy and science', according to the authors who used it as an organizing framework. Within the critical social theory framework, Habermas's (1984) philosophy was adopted. This involved a process of allowing all participants to present their claims as to what they held to be 'truth'. Participatory action research which built on Habermas's philosophy was used to approach the problems and concerns of the CMHNs.

Data collection involved using six focus groups and was followed by report writing and validation. The use of such groups was justified as an effective method by the researchers because they felt that interviewing individuals would be more time-consuming and that a diversity of opinion was important in addressing the problem (Munday, 2006).

Six focus groups were formed to address the nurses' concerns and their recommendations. Focus group participation was voluntary. Group sizes ranged from five to ten people and the duration of the meetings ranged from an hour and a half to two hours. Information was reported while ensuring anonymity and confidentiality were met.

Themes were developed from the focus groups to explain participants' overall concerns conceptualized as a process. A final action plan with implementation steps was drawn up and Task Forces were formed to implement this plan.

Overview of outcomes

Three conceptual outcomes emerged as key concerns for the nurses and formed an umbrella for their recommendations for change. These were: 'Struggling for an Identity and a Collective Voice', 'Valuing Autonomy' and 'Seeking Role Recognition'. The study resulted in a plan of action being developed by the participants to address their concerns.

Researchers' comments on the use of participatory action research

The researchers reported that this study, because of its focus group and PAR methods, empowered the nurses through its processes and that the nurse participants were 'invested in the action plan's outcomes'. Using the PAR framework made the implementation of the interventions and actions more effective. From the researchers' perspective, it was important to have CMHNs participate in a process that would elicit their concerns, a process that was specifically aimed at developing a consensus regarding the expressed concerns and, finally, to assist them in identifying any recommendations for change.

Example 1.3   Hospital mealtimes: action research for change? (Dickinson et al., 2005)

Background

This study was designed to address the problem of poor nutritional care within a hospital setting: specifically to improve the patients' experience of mealtimes. In order to implement patient-centred mealtimes for older patients by changing the focus from institutional convenience to one that focused on their requirements, an action research approach was used that focused on action and change. The project was carried out within a 26-bed unit providing care for older patients with complete discharge needs. Older patients were referred to the unit from throughout the acute NHS Trust, when the acute stage of the

(Continued)

(Continued)

condition that had led to a hospital admission had been stabilised and treated but an immediate return home was not possible because of the resulting frailty and complex diagnosis that necessitated a change in living or care arrangements. Patients generally stayed on the unit for between two weeks and several months.

The aims of the project were to implement patient-focused mealtime practice for older patients within a hospital unit and to promote healthy ageing through improving mealtime care by working towards the implementation of a patient-focused and enabling culture.

The objectives were to work with staff (using an action research approach) to help them to describe and explore the mealtime environment then current on the unit, to explore with staff ways of focusing mealtimes towards the needs of the patients, and to help staff to make changes to the mealtime environment and their practice.

Methods

Qualitative methods were used, which included focus groups, interviews, observations, and benchmarking that utilized the 'Essence of Care' benchmarking tool (Department of Health, 2001). Focus group discussions were held at the beginning of the project, before the action research intervention began, in order to identify any difficulties with mealtimes and nutrition-related work on the unit and this was to be repeated at the end of the implementation phase. The focus group included members of staff working on the unit, together with representation from healthcare assistants, qualified nursing staff, and occupational therapy and physiotherapy staff. Photographs representing mealtimes on the unit were shown to participants as a stimulus to promote a discussion at the beginning of the focus group and the questions used in the groups highlighted various aspects of the mealtime experience. Three focus groups involving 19 staff were undertaken. Qualitative interviews were used to gather detailed in-depth information. The focus was on each individual's experiences and the interviewee was at the centre of this element of the enquiry. Interviews were used to assist with seeing mealtimes from a patient perspective and to explore patients' experiences and views of unit mealtimes. A sample of six patients were interviewed. Observations included the location for eating, the involvement and activity of nursing staff, and the timing and duration of the events; all of these were recorded onto an observational schedule. Data were analysed using interpretive, inductive approaches such as categories, themes, and patterns.

Overview of outcomes

The data fell into three main themes that each impacted on patients' experiences of mealtimes: institutional and organizational constraints, mealtime care and nursing priorities, and the eating environment. When this paper was published, only two of the three phases of the project had been completed. The changes that had been made thus far included alterations to practice at mealtimes that prioritised mealtime care for all staff on the unit, such as making sure that nursing staff were actively involved and had rescheduled other work, e.g. giving out medication, in order to avoid mealtimes. The 'Malnutrition Universal Screening Tool' was also introduced in order to identify those patients at risk of malnutrition, and changes had been made to the physical environment to ensure it was more conducive to mealtimes, including improving the ambience of the dining room by purchasing new crockery and tablecloths, etc.

Researchers' comments on the use of the action research approach

An action research approach was selected by the researchers, as it aims to generate knowledge about social systems as well as attempting to change these (Hart and Bond, 1995). The researchers maintained that by using action research, they were able to improve the mealtime care of patients. They also suggested that the action research approach worked as a vehicle to enable practitioners and researchers to collaborate in their efforts to improve the real world of practice, including the clinical situation and the outcome for patients.

Example 1.4 Time off the ward: an action research approach to reducing nursing time spent accompanying children to X-ray (Beringer and Julier, 2009)

Background

Accompanying children off the ward for radiological and other investigations is a routine part of everyday practice. The medical staff in the location of the project recognized that while such investigations played an important part in childcare, they also found that delays in the process could mean that the child, the family, and the nurse were absent from the ward for longer than was necessary. The aim of the project was to reduce the amount of time nurses spent accompanying children to the X-ray department for radiological investigations. The objectives were to clarify and improve the process of accompanying a child to X-ray and to promote the development of a positive professional relationship with colleagues in the X-ray department.

(Continued)

(Continued)

Methods

An action research approach, based on the cycle of identifying an issue, collecting base-line measures, implementing change, and re-measuring (based on Lewin, 1946) was adopted.

The project was led by a nurse researcher (AB) from the local university, who was funded by the hospital to facilitate a programme of action research projects throughout the Trust. Project meetings started in November 2006 and ran through to March 2008. A total of ten meetings were held. These took place on the ward and at the university.

An audit was carried out to measure the amount of time spent off the ward by nurses accompanying the children over a period of one month. The audit sheet containing such information as the day and time of the event, the grade of staff, their destination, and the duration of absence was completed by staff each time they left the ward. The results were entered into Excel spreadsheets which were then used to analyse the information that had been collected. The analysis was used to highlight the scale of the issue to colleagues and to persuade them that it needed to be addressed. As part of the base-line information gathering the researchers undertook a mapping exercise, using *Post-it* notes to represent all the stages in getting a child to X-ray and to identify the staff involved in each. Using the process map and identifying the staff involved helped the team to recognize that many stages within the process depended on effective communication between the ward and the X-ray department.

Overview of outcomes

An action plan was introduced which included three main measures: to introduce the practice of ward staff telephoning the X-ray department before each visit; to nominate a link nurse to be a professional representative and conduit for communication; to extend the ward orientation programme for new staff members and students so it would include a visit to the X-ray department. These measures were introduced before a second audit was carried out.

The second audit showed that the proportion of time nurses were spending off ward in X-ray had halved since the first audit – from 24 per cent down to 12 per cent. The actual number of hours off the ward had reduced from 52 to 32. It was also found that the key day when most time was spent off the ward had changed from Tuesday to Wednesday. This was useful when preparing the off-duty rota as it enabled the team to anticipate when more staff would be needed. A link nurse from the ward was then identified who made contact with a radiographer from the X-ray department.

Researchers' comments on the use of the action research approach

The facilitated action research approach gave structure and direction to the improvement of this routine aspect of ward practice which provided the team with an opportunity to learn new skills while on the project that they felt could be applied to other situations. Examples of some of these new skills included collecting and processing information and finding the best way to engage with colleagues in different departments to bring about changes to practice, as well as how to make a funding application to support attendance at a conference.

Many of the salient features of action research have been exemplified through these four examples presented above. The context of all the enquiries – healthcare – varies each time. Yet it is evident that for the action researchers involved the ultimate objective of the research enquiry was the production of greater understanding of the selected groups within the system in order to produce practical principles and strategies for the improvement of that system. A possible common denominator for all four action research enquiries was that the population of participants who worked within this healthcare context system were engaged in a collaboration designed to benefit all those involved.

The life courses of participants in the research process seem to have been enhanced. That enhancement may be explained with reference to two elements: a greater understanding of the role of participants in the system founded on more detailed and profound knowledge and a greater understanding of self, due to informed and negotiated meanings of activities shared with others and a developed capacity for construction and analysis.

Summary

In this chapter we have tried to give the reader an overview of what is entailed in carrying out action research and the purposes of carrying out action research projects. The presentation of models and definitions of action research can only give a hint of the flavour of the experience – to digest the nature of action research fully you need to be an active participant. Expert views, from those who have contributed to the development and a more widespread acceptance of action research, were indicated and their names and publications were cited as landmarks in the progress of the methodology. A salient feature of action research is its cyclical structure and this was highlighted by the diagrammatic forms. Different readers will, indeed, react to each diagram differently and use them as they see fit within their own action plans. The key characteristics of the action research approach were explored. Some theoretical underpinnings, associated with action research, were briefly presented. Four examples of previously published action research projects were provided to enable the reader to become acquainted with the various processes and stages prior to experiencing them personally.

Further reading

Blaikie, N. (1993) *Approaches to Social Inquiry*. London: Polity.

Blaxter, L., Hughes, C. and Tight, M. (1996) *How to Research*. Buckingham: Open University Press.

Carr, W. and Kemmis, S. (1986) *Becoming Critical: Education, Knowledge and Action Research*. London: Falmer.

Cohen, L., Manion, L. and Morrison, K. (2007) *Research Methods in Education* (6th edn). London: RoutledgeFalmer.

Creswell, J.W. (2009) *Research Design: Qualitative, Quantitative, and Mixed Methods Approaches*. Thousand Oaks, CA: SAGE.

Elliot, J. (1991) *Action Research for Educational Change*. Buckingham: Open University Press.

Hart, E. and Bond, M. (1995) *Action Research for Health and Social Care*. London: Open University Press.

Hughes, I. (2008) 'Action research in healthcare', in P. Reason and H. Bradbury (eds), *The SAGE Handbook of Action Research: Participative Inquiry and Practice*. London: SAGE.

McNiff, J. and Whitehead, J. (2005) *All You Need To Know About Action Research*. London: SAGE.

Meyer, J. (2000) 'Using qualitative methods in health related action research', *British Medical Journal*, 320: 178–181.

Meyer, J. (2006) 'Action research', in K. Gerrish and A. Lacey (eds), *The Research Process in Nursing*. Oxford: Blackwell.

Reason, P. and Bradbury, H. (2008) *The SAGE Handbook of Action Research: Participative Inquiry and Practice* (2nd edition). London: SAGE.

Stringer, E.T. and Genat, W.J. (2004) *Action Research in Health*. Upper Saddle River, NJ: Pearson Prentice-Hall.

Waterman, H., Tillen, D., Dickson, R. and de Koning, K. (2001) 'Action research: a systematic review and assessment for guidance', *Health Technology Assessment*, 5 (23).

Whitelaw, S., Beattie, A., Balogh, R. and Watson, J. (2003) *A Review of the Nature of Action Research*. Cardiff: Welsh Assembly Government.

Winter, R. and Munn-Giddings, C. (2001) *A Handbook for Action Research in Health and Social Care*. London: Routledge.

2

Engaging in Action Research

This chapter focuses on:

- Types of action research
- Why action researchers choose action research
- The advantages and limitations of action research as a methodology
- The concerns about action research as a research approach
- Action research and professional development
- Action research for managing change
- The processes and outcomes of action research
- Practical examples.

Introduction

In Chapter 1, we discussed some of the definitions and features of action research and considered what makes it a powerful mode of enquiry for practitioners. We tried to establish that the principal aim of carrying out an action research project was to support a researcher or group of researchers in studying an aspect of practice, to study it in-depth, to plan and implement action, and to learn from their experiences. In this chapter we shall explore the different types of action research projects carried out by practitioners and consider why some practitioners engage in action research. We shall also discuss the advantages and the perceived limitations of the action research approach and address the common concerns raised about using it. In addition the role of action research in the professional development of the practitioner is considered. Action research is often described as a means to manage change in healthcare settings. Examples of projects where the change agenda has been achieved are therefore presented and the processes and outcomes involved in action research are considered. In order to facilitate reflection on the latter, a set of practical examples of action research is provided at the end of the chapter.

Before action researchers start a project, whatever their professional context, it would be useful to consider the following two broad questions:

- What are the features of action research which make it a suitable mode of enquiry for practitioners?
- What are the processes involved in carrying out action research?

In this chapter we shall attempt to address these issues and indicate how they apply to action researchers.

In their systematic review of action research Waterman et al. quoted one practitioner's perspective (in a focus group discussion) that outlined the reasons for choosing action research:

> I very much see the world of action research as being something that can take practice forward in a systematic way, while acknowledging the chaos that can be inherent in action research. However, that you are actually impacting on practice … It involves people and you actually make a difference and I think that appeals to me as an individual. I think if I am going to work with practitioners and patients, I want to make a difference. (2001: 21)

Waterman et al. capture the essence of what can be achieved through the use of an action research approach in the context of their study within ophthalmic nursing practice. They state:

> With determination, commitment, and collaboration with patients and other healthcare professionals, we have learnt that we can reverse what was below-standard care to that which we feel able to present at conferences and publish. (2005: 397)

In a powerful endorsement of the use of action research in healthcare contexts, Meyer (2006) describes action research as different to other approaches, as it is centrally concerned with the lessons learnt from practice development, and justifies her stance that in applied disciplines the purpose of research is to understand and improve practice. Meyer argues that while action research can take many different forms and styles, it contributes to common themes of improving practice and implementing change.

First, second and third person research/practice

Reason and Bradbury (2001) offer three broad pathways of action research practice. These are described by the authors as follows:

- First-person action research skills and methods address researchers' ability to foster an inquiring approach to their own lives, to act with awareness and to choose carefully, and to assess the effects in the outside world while acting. First-person research practice brings inquiry into more and more of our moments of action – not as outside researchers but within in the whole range of everyday activities.
- Second-person action research/practice addresses our ability to inquire face-to-face with others into issues of mutual concern, for example in the service of improving our personal and professional practice both individually and separately. Second-person inquiry starts with interpersonal dialogue and includes the development of communities of inquiry and learning organizations.
- Third-person research/practice aims to extend these relatively small-scale projects so that 'rather than defined exclusively as "scientific happenings" they (are) also defined as "political events"' (Toulmin and Gustavsen, 1996). Third-person strategies aim to create a wider community of enquiry involving persons who, because they cannot be known to each other face-to-face (say in a large, geographically dispersed corporation), have an impersonal quality. Writing and other kinds of reporting of the processes and outcomes of inquiries can also be an important form of third-person inquiry.

Reason and Bradbury suggest that the most compelling and enduring kind of action research will engage all three strategies: first-person research practice is best conducted in the company of friends and colleagues who can provide support and challenge; such a company may indeed evolve into a second-person collaborative inquiry process. They add that, on the other hand, attempts at third-person research which are not based in rigorous first-person inquiry into one's purposes and practices are open to distortion through an unregulated bias.

In the context of working with graduate students who choose to adopt a range of first-, second-, and third-person approaches, Reason and Marshall (2001) illuminate the three approaches in practical terms. They state that all good research is *for me, for us,* and *for them.* It is *for them* to the extent that it produces some kind of generalizable ideas and outcomes which can elicit the response 'That's interesting' from those who are concerned with understanding a similar field. It is *for us* to the extent that it responds to concerns for our praxis, both relevant and timely, and so produces the response 'That works' from those who are struggling with problems in their field of action. It is *for me* to the extent that the processes and outcomes respond directly to the individual researcher's being in-the-world and so elicit the response 'That's exciting', taking exciting back to its root meaning, i.e. to set in action.

Types of action research

A close look at the published literature will show that a variety of approaches has been used in carrying out action research. Whitelaw et al. (2003) highlight three broad types of action research in the literature:

- Technical–scientific and positivist.
- Mutual–collaborative and interpretive.
- Critical and emancipatory.

In the following section we will draw on the above explanations of the features of each type supplemented by a commentary from Meyer (2006). We recommend the reader to peruse the original text, which provides examples for each of the types.

Technical-scientific and positivist action research

In this model the action researcher's work would start off with the intention of linking research to action, but would operate within a traditional 'scientific' method. Based on the assumption that experts or those in authority will have greater experience or initial research scope, questions and theoretical resources would be set independent of a significant interaction with the research area and its subjects. These participants act at the level of providing 'on the ground feedback' within fixed parameters. The main aim of the research is to 'test' the effectiveness of a particular pre-defined intervention. Data collection, analysis, interpretation, and ultimate knowledge would be undertaken by researchers. Meyer (2006) suggests that this model is often associated with management consultancy and used extensively by health service managers and that the tendency for a top-down approach endangers ownership of both problems and their solutions by staff.

Mutual-collaborative and interpretivist action research

In this form of action research policy makers, researchers, and field practitioners are perceived as coming together within the context of the research to identify any potential problems, their possible nature, and a range of likely interventions – with the assumption that in an ideal situation of unimpaired communication some form of consensus can be reached. With this model in theory there is consensus and little imposition of authoritarian or expert views, with the prospects for implantation perceived as being high, although Whitelaw et al. highlight that the change can be short-lived as those who are involved in the project leave and are replaced by new individuals with different perspectives. Meyer (2006: 276) does not see this as a problem as she maintains that 'the success of action research does not depend on whether the intended goals are achieved or the change sustained'. She goes on to explain that the intended goals are often linked to policy initiatives and much can be learned from trying to put policy into practice, that it is unrealistic to assume that change will be sustained in ever-changing healthcare contexts. Meyer argues that it takes a long time for new ideas to become embedded in practice.

Critical and emancipatory action research

This third type of action research sees research as an explicit vehicle for political and critical expression. This approach works on the basis that within any system deep-rooted ideological forces will exist that will distort the way that different individuals within it perceive reality and the effects of this will ultimately shape real experiences. Meyer (2006) suggests that this type may not be favoured by funding bodies as it challenges the forces that will profit from maintaining particular viewpoints and values the notions of participation, empowerment, and emancipation. She adds that the majority of literature on action research advocates critical and emancipatory approaches and that the Royal College of Nursing Institute Practice Development Unit also advocates the use of critical and emancipatory approaches to changing practice.

In a different kind of classification, a typology of action research is put forward by Hart and Bond (1995)[1] in which the authors identify four basic types of action research which are: *experimental, organizational, professionalizing* and *empowering*. They propose the following seven criteria to distinguish between the different types of action research. Action research:

1 Is educative.
2 Deals with individuals as members of social groups.
3 Is problem focused, context specific, and future oriented.
4 Involves change intervention.
5 Aims at improvement and involvement.
6 Involves a cyclic process in which research, action, and evaluation are linked.
7 Is founded on a research relationship in which those involved are participants in the change process.

---

[1]Hart, E. and Bond, M. (1995) *Action Research for Health and Social Care*, p. 37. Reproduced with the kind permission of Open University Press.

Why do researchers choose action research in healthcare?

Hughes (2008: 383) observes that making a choice to use action research as an approach for a particular project or purpose may involve:

- having some sense of what it might mean and its potential benefits over other approaches;
- evidence from systematic reviews, research reports, text books, and other literature;
- information from within your organization, internet searches, and non-peer reviewed sources;
- opinions from peers or experts;
- clinical data or other information gathered with clients, families, stakeholders, or co-researchers;
- economic considerations including personnel, equipment, and other resources.

Hughes quotes the five reasons, listed by Waterman et al. (2001), for practitioners choosing action research, based on a review of 48 British reports.

- The most common reasons for choosing AR are concerned with encouraging stakeholders to participate in making decisions about all stages of research, or empowering and supporting participants.
- Frequently cited reasons include solving practical, concrete, or material problems or evaluating change.
- Reasons associated with the research process include contributing to understanding, knowledge, or theory; having a cyclical process included in feedback; or embracing a variety of research methods.
- In some instances action research has been chosen because it educates.
- In a quarter of the studies, it was picked because it acknowledges complete contexts or because it may be used with complex problems in adaptive systems.

Viewpoints from action researchers on why they found the action research approach a useful methodology are included throughout this book. Two particular examples are cited below. First, reporting on a longitudinal study on innovations in health services, Bridges et al. (2007) describe action research as a participatory approach ideally suited to monitoring the process and outcomes of change. Their study reports on how an action researcher looked at the work of four Inter-Professional Care Co-ordinators (IPCCs). The researcher kept regular participant observation field notes and supplemented these data with profiles of 400 IPCCs, in-depth interviews, focus groups with staff, and findings fed back to the participants to inform practice developments. The paper reports on an 'innovative journey' of professions and, in particular, on how such journeys can in fact continue even after their 'end point'.

In the second example, Baron (2009) examines an action research study which involved a patient journey model to improve patient–centred care and the collaboration needed for such a project's success. According to Baron, action research was used:

- as it provided an opportunity to hear patient voices;
- as it enhanced the knowledge, understanding, and inter-professional working practices of those involved;
- as an alternative because 'if surveys and questionnaires were used the results yielded may have indicated only that the patients and their partners/carers were satisfied or very satisfied with their healthcare';
- to help to realize the National Health Service vision of becoming patient-centred, as it was essential that both service users' and service providers' views were taken into account;
- with the clinical data or other information gathered from clients, families, stakeholders, or co-researchers;
- for economic considerations, including personal equipment and other resources.

Advantages and limitations of using action research as a methodology

Utilizing her involvement in practitioner research with teachers, Koshy (2010) lists the unique advantages of using action research as an approach which is applicable in any discipline where research is conducted in practical contexts. Koshy believes that it is a powerful and useful model because:

- research can be set within a specific context or situation;
- researchers can be participants – they don't have to be *distant* and *detached* from the situation;
- it involves continuous evaluation and modifications can be made as the project progresses;
- there are opportunities for theory to emerge from the research, rather than from a previously formulated theory;
- the study can lead to open-ended outcomes.

In the context of using action research in managing and implementing change in healthcare settings, Parkin (2009: 30) summarizes the advantages of the action research methodology.

- It offers a means of solving local problems.
- It promotes an interest in research amongst those not previously involved.
- It defines individuals as active participants rather than passive subjects.
- Group participations help to motivate and maintain interest.

- The focus of the research is meaningful to the participants.
- The results of the research are monitored alongside the actions for rapid feedback.
- It is an acceptable and appropriate method for social and healthcare contexts.
- It encourages self-awareness from both participants and researchers.
- Its results may be able to inform other, similar, contexts and situations.

Parkin also lists the possible limitations of action research, as follows.

- A lack of precision over its nature and definition.
- Potential limitations on generalizing findings beyond the local situation.
- It attracts attendant problems of change management, including resistance and conflict.
- It can be time consuming for little gain.
- It can encounter cultural, professional, and managerial constraints on change initiatives.
- Its methods can conflict with notions of autonomy and individualization particularly where these are highly valued.
- The ethical issues require careful explanation and management.

In this context, Waterman et al's (2001) list of pivotal factors, identified from their systematic review of action research, is a very useful framework for considering the advantages and challenges involved in action research (we recommend the reader look at this section in full for its explanations). The pivotal factors are listed as:

- participation;
- key persons;
- action researcher–participant partnership;
- real world focus;
- resources;
- research methods;
- project process and management;
- knowledge.

Waterman et al. (2001) provide an extensive and very useful list of advantages and disadvantages of action research in their systematic review (again recommended to the reader to examine in full). Meyer (2006: 286) summarizes the key points which can be seen opposite in Table 2.1.

Is action research real research?

Based on a doctoral study seminar with a group of healthcare, social work, and education practitioners – discussing the strengths and limitations or disadvantages in using an action research methodology – Koshy (2010)

TABLE 2.1 *Advantages and disadvantages of action research*

Advantages (*In situations where*)	Disadvantages
• No evidence exists to support or refute current practice.	• Not viewed as science.
	• Findings not generalizable.
• Poor knowledge, skills, and attitudes exist.	• Vulnerability of participants.
• Evidence-based practice needs to be developed.	• Depends on collaboration.
• Gaps have been identified in service provision.	• Difficult to achieve and sustain change
• Services are underused or deemed inappropriate.	• Feedback can be threatening.
• New roles are being developed and implemented.	• Change hard to measure.
• Work is being undertaken across traditional conflicting boundaries.	• Poor development of theory.

argues that when you consider action research for the purposes of professional development or improving a practical situation, it is difficult to accept the many disadvantages listed by those critics of action research. However, the author also acknowledges that action research is sometimes described as a *soft* option by some and recommends that researchers need to define the parameters of a study at the beginning. She addresses four of the main concerns raised by critics.

Concern 1: action research lacks rigour and validity

Questions are sometimes raised on issues about the validity of findings. How can someone achieve objectivity when they are researching their own practice? There are ways of dealing with this. First, they would need to acknowledge their values and epistemological stance right from the start. They could set up a validation group (unless they were working with stakeholders, in which case sharing will be built into the research process) to share the data with before generating evidence and presenting any findings. They would need to be rigorous in both gathering and analysing the data. In action research, the fieldwork is located within someone's own context and practical situation and this should be acknowledged as such. Action researchers are not drawing on national samples of data or organizing randomized controlled trials to assess the effectiveness of a particular drug or treatment. Sharing data with an action research group and triangulation should also ensure that the quality of what is gathered is robust and without bias.

Concern 2: action research findings are not generalizable

The question of generalizability arises in most literature on action research. Koshy (2010) argues that the action researcher does not set out to seek generalizable data, but to generate knowledge based on action within one's own situation. A researcher would be asking: *'What am I doing here?'* and *'How can I improve the situation and my own practice?'*. Any findings from the research are generalizable only within that situation and within the context of the work and the researcher's beliefs, which are declared in advance. The dissemination of findings could be applicable to those who are interested and to other practitioners in similar circumstances, either locally or at a distance. It may also be useful for those who would wish to apply the ideas and findings within similar contexts or to replicate the study.

Concern 3: it is a deficit model

Koshy (2010) maintains that quite often a reference is made to the problem-solving nature of action research which may portray the process as a deficit model. As the research issue or topic arises from researchers' desire to improve practice, the inquiry may not be due to a specific problem. However, if action researchers are trying to solve a problem, developing strategies for solving that problem within a situation is not a negative process! It would effectively be about making progress and developing innovative ideas and strategies.

In their editorial to a special issue of collections of *Action Research* studies, Stringer et al. (2008) state that action research is used by a wide variety of people, from workers to policy makers, to investigate a wide spectrum of issues for a wide range purposes. The authors stress that action research provides the means not only to define more clearly 'what is wrong', namely, to clarify the problematic features of a situation, but also to identify 'what is right', that is, the strengths and assets that provide the base from which to construct effective and sustainable solutions. It is also emphasized here that action research provides the means to assist people with developing the capacity to formulate appropriate, effective sustainable solutions to the complex issues and problems they face and that the rigorous, flexible, and cyclical nature of action research processes can provide a purposeful and meaningful orientation that enables people to make tangible difference to the issues affecting their everyday lives.

Concern 4: action research and mainstream research

In a paper entitled 'How can action research apply to health services?', Morrison and Lilford (2001) identify five key tenets of the action research approach and address the concern of whether action research can be considered scientific (a hotly debated issue) for each of these tenets. A summary of the authors' views can be examined in the following section.

1 *The flexible planning tenet*
The detailed content and direction of a research project are not to be determined at the outset. These take on a definite shape only as the work progresses and are kept continuously under review.

2 *The iterative cycle tenet*
Research activity is to proceed on a cycle of considering what the problem to be researched is, proposing action to resolve that problem, taking action, learning lessons from the result of the action, considering what the problem is in the light of those lessons, and then returning to the cycle again as many times as is necessary. Each phase involves a consultation with all interested parties.

3 *The subjective meaning tenet*
The situational definitions and subjective meanings that those directly implicated in the problem being researched attach to it must be allowed to determine the content, direction, and measures of the success of a research project.

4 *The simultaneous improvement tenet*
A research project must set out to change the problem situation for the better through the very process of researching it.

5 *The unique context tenet*
A research project must explicitly take into account the complex, ever changing, and hence unique nature of the social context in which the project is carried out.

Morrison and Lilford state that proponents of action research are keen to distance it from mainstream research and each of the five tenets carries an implied criticism of mainstream research. They argue that it is as though the proponents are apprehensive that if action research turns out to be unscientific beneath the glare of anyone's spotlight, it will never gain the respectability they believe it merits. Morrison and Lilford take the view that 'they need not take this stance and that it is perfectly respectable to engage in an enquiry, aimed at bringing about beneficial change in a manner sensitive to context, according priority to the perspective of those directly implicated and working iteratively to increase understanding rather than mapping everything out at the start' and hence ask why there is this 'concern about being scientific'.

While Morrison and Lilford do not argue that action research is 'scientific', they believe that some of the five tenets are eminently suitable for health services. They conclude their arguments by stating that:

- action researchers have pioneered a number of practices – flexible planning, the use of iterative cycles, and so on – from which mainstream researchers could profitably learn;
- action researchers deserve much credit for their imagination and initiative in developing these practices and the thinking that underpins them;

- as health services present a highly constrained environment for researchers, some of the ways of working pioneered by action research could, if adopted by mainstream researchers, make their findings more readily useable by the healthcare professions.

Action research and professional development

So what are the salient features of action research that make it a useful methodology for enhancing practitioners' development? A consideration of Carr and Kemmis's (1986) list of what action research entails is a good starting point here. These authors, who are widely cited on action research in healthcare, view action research as an integral part of critical professional development. Although the context of their work is in education, their ideas are relevant and useful within healthcare. Carr and Kemmis list five particular features of action research as a methodology for practitioners. Each of these warrants careful thought and consideration before taking a first step. We have considered some of these ideas in earlier sections of this book, but these are further reinforced here. So what are these five features? First, they assert that action research will entail indicating how it rejects positivist notions of rationality, objectivity, and truth in favour of a dialectical view of rationality. Second, it will entail indicating how action research employs the interpretive categories by using these as a basis for 'language frameworks' which teachers can explore and develop via their own theorizing. Third, action research provides a means by which distorted self-understandings may be overcome by healthcare workers, analysing the way their own practices and understandings are shaped. Fourth is linking reflection to action, offering researchers a way of becoming aware of how those aspects of the social order which frustrate rational change may be overcome. Finally, it involves returning to the question of theory and practice, to show that self-critical communities of action researchers can enact a form of social organization by which truth is determined by the way it relates to practice.

Carr and Kemmis's definition of action research clearly reflects the above sentiments. They maintain that action research is highly relevant to both users and practitioners by stating that action research is:

> a form of enquiry undertaken by participants in social situations in order to improve rationality and justice of their own social or educational practices, as well as their own understanding of these practices and situations in which these practices are carried out. (1986: 162)

Zuber-Skerrit (1996) explains the features of action research as critical and (self-critical) collaborative inquiry by reflective practitioners who are accountable and must make the results of their inquiry public, as well as self-evaluating their practice and being engaged in participatory problem solving and continual professional development.

The all important question to consider here is this: why would a practitioner carry out action research? We can think of several reasons. First, the work of professionals in healthcare is not just about developing a set of technical competencies. The ultimate aim of healthcare work is to enhance the quality of provision for the users. In order to achieve this, in addition to formal qualifications healthcare workers need to attend to their continuing professional development. This can be achieved when practitioners take the time to internalize ideas and this internalization is more likely to be more effective if it is accompanied by reflection. In recent years, the importance of being a reflective practitioner as part of one's professional development has come to the fore for practitioners in all disciplines – for example social workers, teachers and medical workers, to name but a few.

When practitioners are engaged in action research, they are continually evaluating and reflecting on their practice and constructing their own theories based on application. Two of the fundamental aspects of what Schön (1991) describes as the 'reflective practitioner' in the context of education are applicable here. In educational terms, he points out that such professionals (a) stand in control of knowledge rather than being subservient to it and (b) by doing this they are engaged in the process of theorizing and achieving self-knowledge. Winter and Munn-Giddings (2001) reinforce these ideas, as they consider the role of *critical reflection* as an important feature of action research. They believe that one of the critical principles of action research is that the initiator of the research learns about his or her own practice and that consequently action research has become popular as a form of education for professional staff in which learning arises from the process of engaging in practice-based enquiry. They attribute this benefit of action research to the concept of *reflective practice* based on Schön's (1983) emphasis on the continuous reflection required by the complexities and uncertainties of professional practice.

Winter (1996) sees action research as a way of investigating professional experience which links practice and the analysis of practice into a single, continuously developing sequence, while Elliot (1991: 52) states that action research improves practice by developing the practitioner's capacity for discrimination and judgement in particular, complex, human situations' and that 'it unifies inquiry, the improvement of performance and the development of persons into their professional roles'. Groups of professionals who worked on action research projects with the second author of this book often described action research as a constructive inquiry, where the researcher actively and continually constructs knowledge that is based on action. All the examples of action research included in this book bear testimony to the way researchers perceive the benefits of being involved in action research.

In a useful guide to carrying out action research published by the Welsh Assembly Government (2007) the authors stress the benefits of practitioners linking up with academics when carrying out such research. Based on a (2001) study by Dadds and Hart, they list the benefits of action research as follows: it encourages creative thinking by suggesting possibilities for inquiry that might not otherwise be considered; it offers support in weighing up the risks that may be involved and making decisions about their chances of success; and it provides insight into the process of learning to help other practitioners create the best possible conditions for their own learning. One of the most striking features of many of the action research projects led by the second author of this book was the way action researchers rated the opportunities for a co-creation of knowledge that they received with external support from academics. Support from academic partners as listed by these practitioners included: providing directions for searching for and reviewing the existing research literature on a topic; offering training in the research skills of data gathering, analysis, and reflection; and helping with the writing-up of reports and dissemination activities.

In this context, the following description about the processes involved in action research from Reason and Bradbury highlights why being involved in action research enhances professional development:

> since action research starts with everyday experience and is concerned with the development of living knowledge, in many ways the process of inquiry is as important as specific outcomes. Good action research emerges over time in an evolutionary and developmental process, as individuals develop skills of enquiry and as communities of inquiry develop within communities of practice. (2001: 2)

Reason and Bradbury also stress the importance of a continuing dialogue between the members of the action research communities of inquiry which also contributes to the development of professional knowledge:

In a pluralist community of inquiry – whether it be a face-to-face inquiry group, an organization, or community – different individual members are likely to hold different questions with different degrees of interest. Some will be most concerned with relationships, some with action, some with understanding, some with raising awareness. To the extent that dialogue is encouraged between these different perspectives the quality of the inquiry will be increased. We would argue that it is important for the action research team or community of inquiry as a whole, to take time regularly for reflection on the choice-points made along the way and the possible need for re-orientation from time to time. (ibid.: 449)

Action research for managing change

Action research is often used as a means of managing change. In the context of managing change in the National Health Service (NHS) in the UK, Iles and Sutherland (2001) describe action research as a way of using research in an interventionist way, so that the researcher is both the discoverer of problems and solutions and involved in decisions about what is to be done and for what reason. It sees change as a cyclical process where theory guides practice and practice in turn informs theory. In this respect, the authors maintain that that action research puts into practice what Lewin (1946) proposed, that theory should not only be used to guide practice and its evaluation, but that it is equally important that results of evaluation should inform theory in the cyclical process of fact-finding, planning, action and evaluation.

The authors also quote Eden and Huxham (1996) that action research results from the involvement of the researcher with members of an organization over a matter which is of genuine concern to them and in which there is an intent by the organization members to take action based on intervention.

Checkland and Scholes (1999) state that an action research methodology forms the foundation of many approaches to change, with the Soft System Methodology (see Figure 2.1 overleaf) as one such example. A close look at this model shows similarities in the processes with action research.

In an inspiring text on managing change in healthcare using action research, Parkin (2009) states that the primary purpose of action-based research is to bring about change in specific situations, in local systems and realworld environments, with the of aim of solving real problems. As such, Parkin suggests that action research is context bound, that those

Principles

- real world: a complexity of relationships
- relationships explored via models of purposeful activity based on explicit worldviews
- inquiry structured by questioning perceived situation using the models as a source of questions
- 'action to improve' based on finding accommodations (versions of the situation which conflicting interests can live with)
- Inquiry in principle never-ending; best conducted with wide range of interested parties; giving the process away to people in the situation

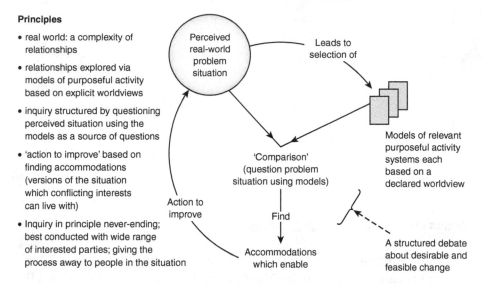

FIGURE 2.1   *The inquiring/learning cycle of the Soft System Methodology (Checkland and Scholes, 1999: 49)*

within the locality participate and collaborate by demonstrating major differences with traditional research. Parkin illustrates the role of action research in managing change with a (2005) study by Leighton that reported on research concerning a mental health rehabilitation unit in the UK that had been designed to assist institutionalized patients with normalizing within society by using a modified therapeutic community approach.

What are the processes and outcomes of action research?

O'Leary describes action research as:

> a strategy that pursues action and knowledge in an integrated fashion through a cyclical and participatory process. In action research, processes, outcome and application are inextricably linked. (2004: 139)

O'Leary also presents the following basic tenets of action research as an approach.

- *It addresses practical problems*
  Action research is grounded in real problems and real-life situations. It generally involves the identification of practical problems in a specific context and an

attempt to seek and implement solutions within that context. As the project is situated within the workplace, ownership of change is a priority and the goal is to improve professional practice. Participatory Action Research often involves the empowerment of the 'marginalized' as they construct their own knowing and attempt to create and action their own strategic plan for emancipation.

- *It generates knowledge*
  Action research is more than just change implementation and relies heavily on both the production of knowledge to produce change and the enacting of change to produce knowledge. Enacting change should not be seen as an end product of knowledge, rather it should be valued as a source of knowledge itself.

- *It enacts change*
  Action research goes beyond knowledge generation and incorporates change into the immediate goals. Whether this is in developing technical skills, building more reflexive professional development or emancipation and liberation, action research works towards a situation improvement that is based in practice.

- *It is participatory*
  In action research, researchers collaborate with practitioners and other stakeholders. Contrary to many other research paradigms, action research works *with* rather than *on* or *for* the researched and is therefore often seen as embodying democratic principles. A high value is placed on local knowledge.

- *It is a cyclical process*
  Action research is a cyclical process that takes shape as knowledge emerges. Cycles converge towards a better situational understanding and improved action implementation and are based in evaluative practice that alternates between action and critical reflection. The goal is to continuously refine methods, data, and interpretation in light of the understandings developed in earlier cycles.

Here is a task for the reader. When reading the examples of action research presented in the next section, try to consider to what extent the selected project involves the basic tenets put forward by O'Leary (2004). Writing thoughts down would be helpful, while working with a colleague or a team and discussing what each of the items means would enhance reader understanding.

The four examples of action research given below demonstrate the varied types and nature of projects conducted by healthcare professionals. Although the accounts are presented in a summary form, we have tried to include all the salient points and messages by presenting these as closely as possible to the original published papers. Reading the papers in their entirety is recommended and full references are provided in the references section. These should exemplify many of the aspects of action research discussed in this chapter.

Example 2.1   Introducing a post-fall assessment algorithm into a community rehabilitation hospital for older adults (Fenton, 2008)

Background

Falls are a significant and frequent occurrence for older adults in community hospitals and are the commonest reportable incident in hospitals, posing major risks to patients who suffer them and to health care organizations (National Patient Agency, in Oliver et al., 2000). At the South Birmingham Primary Care Trust, normal practice for the assessment of patients following a fall was varied because nurses did not assess patients in a standard manner and usually contacted a doctor immediately for their attendance whether the patient was injured or not. The project was designed to develop a new assessment tool to guide nurses in the evaluation of patients following a fall. The idea behind the assessment tool was that it would support nurses in prioritizing medical attendance to review particular patients by requesting immediate, same day, or next working day care.

Methodology

An action research approach was used to change clinical practice. This approach was selected as it was felt to be effective in the implementation of change in a clinical environment, involving collaboration and re-education and changing ways of thinking.

A multi-disciplinary focus group of eight members, including a physiotherapist, occupational therapist and a wide representative of grades – selected for their interest and expertise in falls assessment and treatment – met a total of six times over three months. They applied a cyclic approach of fact finding, planning, taking action, and evaluating to refine and develop the tool. The group met a further three times to develop the tool and prepare for its trial on an inpatient rehabilitation ward for older people; another two subsequent meetings were necessary to review the feedback from ward staff on the use of the tool and one more took place to evaluate and finalize the project. Data collection was a continuous process from focus group discussions and comments from ward staff. After each meeting all the participants received meeting notes to check for accuracy and a correct representation. A sample of 15 patients was reviewed during the trial of the post-fall algorithm (the tool in question) using an audit form.

Overview of outcomes

Fenton reported that the post-fall assessment algorithm developed during the project could be used by staff in other clinical areas for patients who had fallen. Staff required only brief training in the use of the algorithm and found it a useful prompt. The algorithm improved decision making regarding requesting attendance of the doctor. The focus group concluded that the post-fall assessment algorithm should be rolled out on all other wards in the community hospitals, form part of the falls prevention policy, and be added to the computerized incident report system.

Researchers' comments on the use of action research methodology

A technical and collaborative action research approach was applied to this project, in which the researcher had a pre-determined agenda and sought collaboration for the development and implementation of the intervention (Holter and Schwartz-Barcott, 1993). Although the participants had had no previous experience of research, they could relate to action research methodology and during the initial development meetings there was a 'transition of ownership' of the tool from the author/researcher to the group.

The action research methodology was appropriately applied to creating and sustaining change in clinical practice by using the key principles of action research – collaboration, empowerment, and participation.

Example 2.2   Encountering the culture of midwifery practice on the postnatal ward during action research: an impediment to change (McKeller et al., 2009)

Background

The reduction of time available to midwives during the hospital postnatal stay suggested there was a need to review postnatal care. It was felt that innovative strategies were required which could give special attention to specific family needs to assist in the transition to parenthood. The aim of the project was to enhance the provision of postnatal care to parents in the early postnatal period, given the time constraints in place for each woman's hospital stay.

The actions were designed to enhance the preparation of parents for parenthood. These included a postnatal planner booklet, a brochure for mothers, and information postcards for fathers. The actions were developed with input from parents via focus group discussions and telephone interviews.

(Continued)

(Continued)

Methodology

Action research was used to explore the educational experiences of parents in the postnatal period. An action research group (ARG) was established, with midwives being predominant members of the group. Data were collected from parents through questionnaires, focus groups and interviews. Three actions were developed and implemented in the postnatal ward.

The actions were evaluated by 122 parents through self-report questionnaires. Midwives working on the postnatal ward and midwives in the ARG provided feedback regarding these actions via separate focus group and group discussions.

Overview of outcomes

The parents who participated in the study and the midwives in the ARG were positive about the actions and perceived them to be beneficial in preparing parents for parenthood. Many of the ward midwives, however, were negative about the actions and questioned their benefit for midwifery practice.

The ways in which midwives in the action research group and the ward midwives reacted were very different. According to McKeller et al., 'the negativity of the ward midwives regarding the innovations implemented in the study contrasted strikingly with the more positive responses from both parents and the ARG midwives'. Possible reasons for this are suggested in the paper.

Two themes which emerged suggested possible reasons for the midwives' responses to the actions – a lack of ownership of the actions and the problematic nature of the culture of a postnatal care environment.

Researchers' comments on selecting action research methodology

An action research methodology with cycles of planning action, observation, and reflection was selected. This approach was chosen because it provided a democratic, collaborative, and dynamic framework for the inquiry. The aim was to improve practices and involve people in the process of change. While the study highlighted some difficulties, it also provided useful insights and ideas for further research.

Example 2.3 Making diabetes education accessible for people with visual impairment (Williams, 2009)

Background

The purpose of this study was to identify any changes that were necessary to make diabetic education materials and the programmes of the Diabetic

Association of Greater Cleveland (DAGC) more accessible for people who had a visual impairment and diabetes (PVID). The DAGC was a local, voluntary, nonprofit diabetic association. Its mission was 'to improve the lives of people affected by diabetes by leading the Northeast Ohio Community in its prevention, management and cure'. Its activities included the support of local diabetic research and the education both of the general public and health professionals. The research question for this study was: What changes are needed to make Diabetic Self Management Education (DSME) materials and programmes accessible for people with visual impairment and diabetes?

Methods

The methodology for his project was Participatory Action Research (PAR) defined as an approach based on collaborative problem solving between researchers and clients which aimed to solve the problem and generate new knowledge. Williams stressed the democratic, equitable, and empowering nature of the process and the importance of including the participation of all stakeholders as equally valuable human beings. The research adopted Stringer's (1999) Look-Think-Act framework: the *look* phase to gather information; the *think* phase as the time for explaining, analysis, interpreting, and explaining; and the *act* phase for planning, implementing, and evaluating any changes.

For this project five visually impaired participants (VIPs) who all had diabetes and four staff members of DAGC worked together (with the author-researcher) as a Planning Group to make DAGC's self-published patient education material and community patient education programmes accessible. The five participants, who had participated in a previous project, were invited to become members of a focus group for this project .

After the initial meeting, the Planning Group met once a month for a year. At each meeting, the group *looked* by reviewing progress since the last meeting and reported new information about needs or resources, *thought* by discussing reports and new information, and planned *acting* by setting the goals for work to be done before the next meeting. Other meetings included recording printed information at a recording station and at one of these the DAGC staff provided an in-service presentation. Transport was organized for those VIPs who were unable to drive and larger print or audio information was made available at the beginning and end of each meeting. Evaluation was a continuous process and a qualitative evaluation was also organized at the end of the project.

Overview of outcomes

Four transformational points and brief comments about the importance of the events in the collaborative process were recorded along with a summary of the steps that the DAGC took as a result of the project to increase accessibility. Changes made to increase accessibility included the production of recordings

(Continued)

(Continued)

to provide access to print information about diabetes; planning the publicity for a public education programme and the locations for accessing this; developing guidelines to help speakers make their diabetes education presentations accessible for people who could not see slides and gestures; and presenting an in-service session for the entire staff of the diabetes association that would include information about how they live with a visual impairment and the common courtesies that made communications with PVID more effective.

Researchers' comments on selecting action research methodology

The researchers felt that PAR gained its power through the story of how the participants grew to understand each other (Greenwoood and Levin, 1998). They also maintained that the PAR report helped readers to have an empathetic understanding of the 'lived reality' of the participants and that focusing on 'epiphanic events' in the PAR process – those turning points that had the power to be 'transformational' – was a way to communicate with reality (Stringer, 1999).

Example 2.4   Participatory action research in the training of primary healthcare nurses in Venda (Van Deventer and Hugo, 2005)

Background

With a strong emphasis on primary healthcare in the health system in South Africa since the 1980s, it became important to ensure relevant skills in rural areas. The authors became aware of problem-orientated learning and patient and community centredness during research on family medicine in light of the fact that community involvement in health was of tremendous value although difficult to attain. Therefore the process of training was examined with the assistance of nursing students who were undertaking a one-year Primary Health Care (PHC) diploma. The aim of the study was for the authors to understand and be part of a process of change in the training of PHC nurses in Venda. Three interrelated themes kept emerging during the research: participatory action research, community development, and learning.

Methods

It was recognized that the project should be a partnership of people who could examine the happenings around them together and their significance. In practice, the ten nursing students doing the PHC course were the unit of analysis and all others (e.g. community members, board members of the PHC Education Unit, and various others) were kept informed of the process.

During the one-year diploma, the nursing students and trainers visited the rural villages, distributed a survey, and held on-going meetings with community members in the villages. The students themselves chose the particular grouping of three villages lying in a valley – these were situated in a very isolated area. Practical experience of communicating with the villagers and developing an understanding of their needs were to become an important part of the nursing students' learning experience.

A simple 'listening survey' was conducted in which one open question was asked: 'What is happening here in this village?' This was followed by seven meetings with the villagers, over the year that the PHC training took place, to give feedback about what had been said by them and to work with them towards some sort of resolution of their problems. One of the students facilitated the meeting in a local language. After this took place, the students and their facilitator returned to the hospital and together reflected on the minutes. This reflection was then documented in a diary form. Qualitative methods were used to understand the nurses' perceptions of the training process. The 'new' knowledge being created was then utilized for the curriculum of the next cycle of nurse training.

Six months after the nurse training was completed, a focus group and two discussion groups were held by the trainer/researcher. The nurses were asked the question: 'What happened for you during the year that we were meeting with M?' (M was the name given to the collective villages). Further clarification and facilitation then followed. The focus group was videotaped and other small group discussions were summarized in a written form.

Overview of outcomes

During the initial survey a number of needs were mentioned by the community members. A week after their survey a meeting was held with the headman of M village who indicated that there was no clinic and if one was built all other things would follow; e.g. telephones and roads. During several meetings with the community two lists were created: the community's perceived needs (electricity, a sports ground, a reliable primary healthcare team, pure water) and the PHC nurses' perceptions of needs (personal hygiene, eye problems, clinic accessibility, care groups). After each visit the students were asked to write about the processes. The issues raised included: the open nature of the discussion with the villagers and their 'good' feelings after sharing the problems (though solving these posed challenges and required the building of relationships). Although it was not part of the aim of the action research study a clinic was built and was functioning using donations.

The results showed that the students felt both empowered and disempowered by the experience. They found it easier to communicate with the communities

(Continued)

(Continued)

they went back to after their training and some problem-based research was spontaneously undertaken by trainees who had been part of the nurse training programme with clinic attenders. However, the nurses also experienced a great deal of resistance from the healthcare system. They felt powerless to help their own communities because of a feeling that they could not gain enough access to financial decision making. New knowledge that emerged showed a need to reflect regularly on the learning process and to be conversant in the vocabulary of family medicine and community development.

Researchers' comments on action research

The researchers felt that in the process of action research there was 'much significant learning acquired through "doing". This is facilitated when "the students participate responsibly" and "when the subject matter is perceived by the student as having relevance to his own purposes.' The participants felt there was responsibility and relevance, as well as self-directed learning and facilitation, rather than just a lecture on the process that had been followed.

The authors felt that working with these communities needed a commitment to a certain worldview, namely one that accommodated the participation of all role players, that understood learning as an experimental process, and that could see the value of community-based research.

As a result of this exposure to the dynamic of rural villages, some directly-related feelings of empowerment were experienced. The nurses also felt that they had gained respect for the opinions of rural non-professional people.

The potential of storytelling was also recognized. The time-line given to the villagers to do things was presented as a story rather than a chart. They felt that whilst a time-line concentrated on the past and present a story could also react with the future and this was felt to be a promising way to harness hope and change.

Summary

This chapter focused on the enhancing qualities of conducting action research. We explored the different types of action research and considered why researchers chose action research as an approach. We considered the advantages and the perceived possible limitations of action research as a methodology and then tried to address some of the criticisms leveled against action research and explained its purpose in terms of improving practice. A case was made for carrying out action research by highlighting its value for educational and professional enhancement. The five features of action research proposed by Carr and Kemmis were presented. Although these may appear complex, they do provide the essence of what is involved in the search for truth, through action research, and should steer the reader towards the practical benefits for healthcare workers. The reader was also introduced to O'Leary's indicators of the structure and processes involved in action research and was invited to consider these within the four practical examples of action research projects that were presented.

Further reading

Carr, W. and Kemmis, S. (1986) *Becoming Critical: Education, Knowledge and Action Research*. London: Falmer.

Cohen, L. and Manion, L. (1994) *Research Methods in Education*. London: Routledge.

Creswell, J.W. (2009) *Research Design: Qualitative, Quantitative, and Mixed Methods Approaches*. Thousand Oaks, CA: SAGE.

Dadds, M. and Hart, S. (2001) *Doing Practitioner Research Differently*. London: Routledge Falmer.

Elliot, J. (1991) *Action Research for Educational Change*. Buckingham: Open University Press.

Hart, E. and Bond, M. (1995) *Action Research for Health and Social Care*. London: Open University Press.

Hughes, I. (2008) 'Action research in healthcare', in, P. Reason and H. Bradbury (eds), *The SAGE Handbook of Action Research: Participative Inquiry and Practice*. London: SAGE.

Lingard, L., Albert, M. and Levinson, W. (2008) 'Grounded theory, mixed methods, and action research', *British Medical Journal*, 337: 459–461.

Meyer, J. (2000) 'Using qualitative methods in health related action research', *British Medical Journal*, 320: 178–181.

Meyer, J. (2006) 'Action research', in, K. Gerrish and A. Lacey (eds), *The Research Process in Nursing*. Oxford: Blackwell.

Morrison, B. and Lilford, R. (2001) 'How can action research apply to health services?', *Qualitative Health Research*, 11(4): 436–449.

O'Leary, Z. (2004) *The Essential Guide to Doing Research*. London: SAGE.

Parkin, P. (2009) *Managing Change in Healthcare: Using Action Research*. London: SAGE.

Reason, P. and Bradbury, H. (2008) *The SAGE Handbook of Action Research: Participative Inquiry and Practice* (2nd edition). London: SAGE.

Stringer, E.T. and Genat, W.J. (2004) *Action Research in Health*. Upper Saddle River, NJ: Pearson Prentice-Hall.

Waterman H., Tillen, D., Dickson, R. and de Koning, K. (2001) 'Action research: a systematic review and assessment for guidance', *Health Technology Assessment*, 5(23).

Welsh Assembly Government (2007) *Action Research Resource Pack*. Available at www.wales.gov.uk/cmoresearch

Whitelaw, S., Beattie, A., Balogh, R. and Watson, J. (2003) *A Review of the Nature of Action Research*. Cardiff: Welsh Assembly Government.

Winter, R. and Munn-Giddings, C. (2001) *A Handbook for Action Research in Health and Social Care*. London: Routledge.

3

Reviewing Literature

This chapter focuses on:

- The purpose of reviewing relevant literature
- Stages in carrying out a literature review
- The sources of literature
- Evaluating sources from the internet
- Organizing and managing your literature review
- Reviewing and writing up the literature.

Introduction

In this chapter we shall focus on the process of undertaking a review of the literature that relates to the topic of a study. As a researcher, the reader will need to be aware of what others have discovered about aspects related to the topic of inquiry and consider how their findings relate to what the reader is about to study. In order to achieve this the reader will need to search and locate a suitable range of literature and analyse and review the different types of studies identified via this search. Researchers can often find the process of undertaking a literature review quite challenging, because it may take hours of work in the library or on the internet which can generate a vast amount of literature that can be quite overwhelming. However, as is the case with all aspects of conducting research, by systematically working and giving careful thought to our efforts this can be made manageable. This process can certainly enhance the reader's understanding of the different strands of an investigation.

Punch (2009) states that the purpose for reviewing literature is to establish what previous empirical evidence there is about a research question and what that evidence tells us. He quotes Fink's (2005: 3) definition (which comes from a book written expressly for researchers in medicine and health): *A research literature review is a systematic, explicit and reproducible method for identifying, evaluating and synthesising the existing body of completed and recorded work produced by researchers, scholars and practitioners.*

Literature reviewing in action research

First we must address an important question which is often posed by action researchers: if the aim of an action research project is to set up structures to improve a local situation, does it matter what other people have found out? The answer to this question will emerge powerfully in the following sections of this chapter, but here is a brief explanation. Undertaking a literature review should enable action researchers to gain insights into the topic for study and consider different perspectives, which in turn, can enhance their confidence in both undertaking the study and disseminating the findings, whether this is in the form of a written or website report, a dissertation, a conference publication, or journal articles. It is also worth remembering that when undertaking an action research inquiry, knowledge of the literature can continue to inform us when making adjustments and refinements throughout a study. Although the reasons for undertaking a literature review in action research are mostly the same as in all research, the process may vary according to the nature of the participant groups and the scope of the inquiry. For example, when conducting action research, a preliminary search and review of related literature might be carried out by the lead researcher or facilitator (who may an academic) with the findings then discussed with the participating group of researchers. The second author of this book has often encouraged teacher researchers to undertake some group or paired readings of literature and to then highlight any key findings followed by a discussion with the larger group of researchers.

While for practical purposes we have included the process of reviewing literature within a defined sequence in the action research process in Chapter 4, it is worth remembering that a review of related literature can support all stages of action research. A good researcher will start reading about a topic as soon as an idea is being considered for inquiry. In the context of carrying out action research, undertaking a literature review can help a researcher to focus on a topic or research question, support their rationale for undertaking the study, help select an appropriate methodology, and aid in structuring the discussions and the final writing-up. As O'Leary (2004: 66) points out, the 'production of new knowledge is fundamentally dependent on past knowledge' and 'it is virtually impossible for researchers to add to a body of literature if they are not conversant with it'. O'Leary's following assertion provides an appropriate background to this chapter:

> ... working with literature is an essential part of the research process. It inspires, informs, educates and enlightens. It generates ideas, helps form significant questions, and is instrumental in the process of research design. It is also central to the process of writing-up; a clear rationale supported by literature is essential, while a well-constructed literature review is an important criterion in establishing researcher credibility.

The purpose of a literature review

A literature review serves the purpose of providing researchers with authoritative support, guidance, and explanations on the topic for inquiry. By reviewing other researchers' findings, they can share their research journeys and experiences and through this process new and previously uncharted territory or new directions could be illuminated. In the context of carrying out action research projects, we surmise researchers would be undertaking a literature review for the following specific purposes:

- To find out what other researchers have unearthed previously about the topic of interest. By considering the key ideas generated by others in the field and the theories developed by other researchers and practitioners in the context of healthcare, they could become familiar with ideas generated not only through action research projects, but also through other types of research. For example, if the purpose of a study is to make improvements in a general practice by setting up support for patients requiring blood sugar control for diabetes, it is important that both the facilitators and the group of researchers update their knowledge about research findings in that field, as well as search for studies in which action researchers have undertaken research with a similar purpose.
- An effective search and review of existing literature can help researchers to become familiar with the terminology, key ideas, and the interconnected nature of different aspects surrounding the topic for research.
- It should help researchers to decide whether a line of inquiry is appropriate and feasible. This is not to discourage them from pursuing a topic of study which has been researched before, on the assumption that 'there is no need to reinvent the wheel'. If researchers find a similar study to the one they are about to undertake, they may decide to replicate it within their own context using an appropriate set of methods. This may help them assess whether a set of findings generated from a different study could be applicable to their own context. Whatever the outcome of the research, everyone needs reminding that the action researcher generates knowledge within a professional context as part of continuing professional development.

Here are some more reasons why a literature search and review could help in action research. Getting to know the literature relating to a study should:

- help researchers to identify what has been done before. In the context of carrying out action research, it is not a just a matter of considering whether there are identifiable gaps in previous research findings, this also helps to ground ideas within the existing literature;
- help researchers develop a conceptual understanding of the topic of inquiry by connecting ideas with insights gained from previous research findings;
- provide researchers with the academic vocabulary used within the topic;
- provide a background to the inquiry and help researchers to articulate a rationale for the study, making adjustments if necessary;
- support researchers in reviewing and refining the research topic, question or hypothesis;
- enable researchers to locate the project within current debates and viewpoints;
- provide a backcloth and framework for the study;
- help researchers to develop research skills to analyse findings and discuss these with rigour and scholarship.

While it is good to read as much as possible about your topic of study, researchers also need to be realistic in terms of what can be managed. It is also helpful to consider what is expected. Again, researchers' personal circumstances will have some bearing on the decision as to the extent of a literature search.

If researchers are carrying out action research as part of an accredited study such as a Master's or doctoral programme, they will be expected to present a comprehensive review of the literature and to demonstrate their understanding of the issues surrounding a topic. The research literature should help build up a framework for the fieldwork required. It should also provide a basis for any further discussion of issues after the data have been collected and analysed. Researchers would need to ask how their data relate to the findings and theories put forward by others.

If researchers are undertaking a small-scale action research project as part of a local initiative, they would still need to read up about the topic as it would help to contextualize the study within the existing literature. In this case researchers may want to focus on a smaller number of key readings. So, to summarize, action researchers need to undertake a literature search and analysis in order to understand, locate, plan, and evaluate a study more effectively.

Stages in carrying out a literature review

As is the case in all aspects of conducting research, it may be useful for researchers to consider the different stages in undertaking a literature review, although they may find that these overlap and might not always follow a pre-determined direction or progression. Also, as previously mentioned, the nature of the literature review will vary according to the nature of the project in terms of its scope, the period of study, and the specific purpose of carrying out the study. The different stages are:

- locating suitable sources;
- organizing and managing the literature;
- reading and appraising the literature;
- reviewing and writing up any readings.

We will discuss each of these stages in sequence.

Locating suitable sources

First, what are the sources of the literature? If researchers are studying for an academic course or working with a facilitator from an academic institution, they will be given a reading list with key readings and information. University-based research and development centres and their websites can also provide helpful sources of recent information. They will publicize conferences and seminars which may be of interest, allowing the opportunity to listen to experts in the field that is being researched. Health journals and newspapers can also provide information on conferences and courses which researchers may wish to attend.

Most libraries will have good systems in place for accessing literature in the form of books and journals; research papers can also be accessed electronically using key word searches. The different sources include: papers published in professional and refereed journals; papers published on the internet; books; the websites of professional associations; the media; and, increasingly, blogs and podcasts. Hard copies of papers can be accessed from a library and abstracts of papers can help researchers decide whether the findings are worth further consideration. Dissertations from Master's and doctoral students are also useful sources, especially in terms of the extensive list of references they can provide. Studies carried out using an action research approach will be particularly useful, as these can provide guidance on the use of this methodology and its associated benefits and the possible challenges experienced by other researchers.

A search through the literature is bound to generate such a large amount of information that anyone may be overwhelmed by it all. This is partly as a result of the internet age we live in and the facilities now available for fast information retrieval. What this requires is to skim read to find out what is being offered and to then select a few sources which are directly relevant to the topic under inquiry.

Before embarking on a search for literature relating to a topic, the following step-by-step suggestions may prove helpful:

- In the initial search – especially if this is on the web - researchers are likely to find a large number of books, chapters in books, journal papers, and newspaper articles. They should aim to select some key readings within the topic. Finding existing papers, which have reviewed the topic of interest is a good start. If someone is studying for an accredited course, consulting a supervisor and some colleagues first and taking their advice may be of benefit. If the work relates to a new policy initiative, then a researcher must look at government websites and listings of current conference presentations. Trying to get a balance of books and papers is always a good idea. Publishers are likely to publish key texts on various topics for current research. It is best to select refereed papers published in peer-reviewed journals, as these go through rigorous quality procedures.

- Faced with a large number of references to select from, how do researchers whittle the numbers down to a manageable amount? A practical suggestion is that they select related literature published within seven to ten years and read this, although this may not always be possible if there is no available literature published recently. Researchers may find that some key sources relating to the historical context of the topic and other significant research findings from the past will be referenced within these papers. These can then be tracked down as necessary and reviewed. It is important to conduct a comprehensive review of theory and research on the subject under inquiry as researchers are seeking 'expertise' status in the field.

- A frequently asked question from researchers is this: how many references do I need? There is no simple answer here. It depends on the nature of the inquiry, the nature of the award-bearing course they are studying for, and how much published literature is available on a subject. The only point we would stress is that whatever the time-scale of research, those undertaking it must show that they are aware of the important developments in the topic of inquiry. Researchers should also be aware of any landmark papers in a particular field.

Sources of literature

There are two main sources of literature available. *Primary sources* include research monographs, government publications, reports, policy documents, research papers, dissertations, conference presentations, and institutional occasional papers with accounts of research. *Secondary sources* use primary sources as references, such as papers written for professional conferences and journals, books written for practising professionals, and book reviews. Reading secondary sources can often give a researcher a feel for a topic. Both types of literature can be located by searching through the websites of specialist and professional organizations, the websites of academic journals, and research conferences.

There are various forms of literature that need consideration. The following sections look at a selection.

Policy related documents

This includes official documents which outline policies within healthcare, which the practitioner needs to be familiar with. These should be available from government websites, published reports, and the libraries of health-care institutions. If a research topic is to do with recent guidelines on patient care, reading the relevant official documents will help researchers to understand the rationale and context of an initiative. The rationale pro-vided in these official documents – often justified in terms of theory and research – may spark some new ideas. Papers may also address the issues around new initiatives in current professional journals. Recent newspaper articles can also often provide insights into new policy initiatives and developments. These insights can be useful when setting up the context or background for work.

Journal articles

A vast amount of research literature is available in research journals relating to healthcare which can be accessed electronically. These can range from large-scale studies to the findings from small-scale action research projects carried out by other researchers. It is often very useful to read about others' research findings and also to take note of the methodology they have used, especially if the researchers have used action research as their approach. These can support a researcher with a choice of methods for data gathering and analysis. It is worth making a critical appraisal of the methodology used by others. Asking whether the data-gathering methods (see Chapter 5) were appropriate is helpful and were the data analysed effectively? Are the find-ings validated and presented clearly and coherently (see Chapter 6)? Starting with the most recent of these sources is worthwhile. Websites of subject associations, professional organizations and government research sites can prove useful sources.

The Cochrane Library

The Cochrane Library is produced by the Cochrane Collaboration which is an international organization. It provides systematic research reviews on different topic areas including healthcare interventions. It also contains the databases for CENTRAL which provides details of randomized trials; this is a rich source of information for researchers.

Research reports

In addition to published papers, a search for research reports can prove useful to researchers. Some of these reports may deal with studies which employed an action research approach. It is possible that a report obtained from the internet has also been published as a journal paper, but the full report should give more details of the research methods used as well as further references to related studies. As in all cases, researchers need to address issues of quality. Databases such as the Health Management Information Consortium would be good places for conducting a search of relevant literature.

Using electronic databases

Various electronic databases can also provide a researcher with a range of literature. Searching can encompass several criteria with 'key words', 'Author', 'Title', and so on. By using key words this is still likely to generate a larger number of sources of literature, but by narrowing the option the number of sources can be reduced. When these have been generated, the next step is reading the abstracts – short summaries of the content of the source – which can provide an overview of the findings. If the abstract looks useful, then accessing the full version of the paper could be worthwhile. Using electronic databases can be challenging and requires acclimatization and practice, so it may be useful for a researcher to work first with someone who has used it before. A library will the best place here to visit for support. Researchers may also wish to look at journal websites for references and abstracts which are also included in the electronic databases.

In the internet age we live in, it is not surprising that this is one of the most useful sources of information. Healthcare workers can access all the major electronic databases and journals. There are several search engines available, with the National Healthcare Library one such example. Professional groups such as the Royal College of Nursing also provide access to healthcare-related journals for their members. International databases such as Google, Google Scholar, MSN, and Yahoo can be searched for research on specific topics by using key words. Healthcare-related international databases include:

- CINAHL (the Cumulative Index to Nursing and Allied Health), which has references to a large set of healthcare journals, conference proceedings and reports;
- MEDLINE, which provides a very large database (with over 12 million records) covering various medical topics;
- EMBASE, which covers health-related papers with a particular coverage in Europe;
- AMED, which provides a database of allied and complimentary medicines;
- The Cochrane Library (as mentioned earlier).

Evaluating sources from the internet

When accessing literature directly from the internet, researchers will need to evaluate the information they retrieve very carefully. As the internet provides us with a large range of sources of information, one needs to be aware of ways of evaluating these. Giving a comprehensive list of evaluating criteria is beyond the scope of this book, so we would recommend the reader look at O'Dochartaigh's (2007) chapter on the evaluation of internet sources and how to assess their credibility and authority. For the benefit of any beginning researchers, we are including a set of guidance notes here, based on O'Dochartaigh's book, which the reader may wish to consider:

- Does the material belong to advocacy groups? If this is so, it is possible that their purpose is to advocate a specific viewpoint or cause. Whilst many such groups do produce work of a very high quality and integrity, in some cases while in pursuit of the advancement of a particular point of view the sources may exaggerate claims and distort views. Researchers need to be careful when citing these in their research. Searching for alternate views which should also be on the web is recommended here.
- As the academic papers which are published in refereed journals are subject to peer reviews, these will probably be a first option for researchers. Papers published on university websites are also subject to quality procedures. But it is worth remembering that there are also many papers which can be accessed on websites that have been included by the authors themselves and that describe their own viewpoints. As these have not always been subject to any reviewing procedures, researchers need to be careful when making use of these without a careful appraisal.
- Although it is important to be aware of up-to-date debates and developments researchers need to employ some caution when reviewing newspaper and magazine articles accessed from the web. News items can often take a certain political point of view. The emphasis on content (articles and stories) is likely to depend on the editorial position taken and as a reviewer a researcher will need to be aware of this. Considering the objectivity of what is published in these outlets before accepting the literature is a worthwhile option.

The reader may wish to consider the following questions, taken from the criteria for an evaluation of internet sources by O'Dochartaigh:

- Is it clear who is responsible for the document?
- Is there any information about the person or organization responsible for the page?
- Is there a copyright statement?
- Does it have a print counterpart that reinforces its authority?
- Are any sources clearly listed so they can be verified?
- Is there any editorial input?
- Are the spelling and grammar correct?
- Are the biases and affiliations clearly stated?
- Are there dates available for when the document was last updated or revised?

Organizing and managing the literature

Organizing the literature

One of the challenges facing researchers is organizing all the literature that is gathered. This needs to be systematic in all aspects of managing a literature review. If a researcher has gathered a good range of literature on a topic the challenge then is to organize the collection and make it manageable and useful. It is useful to bear in mind that a researcher will also need to access any reading at the time of writing-up. Being meticulous about keeping a record of what is being read in terms of references to the texts or articles is important. Summaries of what has been read are useful. A number of our students have told us that they wished they had been more organized with their collection of literature. Many of them will read and think about the content and will then store paper copies in box files, thinking that they can go back and find the relevant references when they need them. This strategy can prove inefficient and result in wasting a lot of time. As one reads more, the more difficult and more chaotic it can become. And sometimes it can also become very frustrating and time-consuming when trying to track down the references as they are required!

Organizing a literature search efficiently from the start is vital, although this may sound like stating the obvious. Here is one practical suggestion using an example from a research topic – patient engagement in ways of controlling pain in osteoarthritis. Suppose a researcher managed to get two journal articles from the library and some printouts of the outline of a project relating to this topic from a website. Assume they also obtained a printout of a summary of an initiative from a government website or a set of clinical guidelines. After reading its contents the researcher decided to send for the whole document. A further search on the web generated more recent references on this particular topic in professional newsletters and a newspaper. Now the researcher had several references to manage and store.

Managing the literature

As researchers will need to retrieve the references they have managed to access and read at different stages of their action research, it is important they set up a system which can enable them to do this right from the start. If they are engaged in a small-scale project one of the simple and traditional ways of organizing all these sources of information is for researchers to do this manually by recording the key information on index cards. They would need to record the title of the book, chapter or paper, the author, date, nature of the content, and a short commentary, including any direct quotes they may wish to put in at a later date. Two simple examples are illustrated below.

Example 1

Authors: A. Grant and M. Robling (2006)

Title: Introducing undergraduate medical teaching into general practice: an action research study

Source and details: Medical Teacher, 28 (7): 192–197

Notes

The study found having medical students in the practice gave members of the primary healthcare team an enhanced sense of worth and made them feel more confident in their professional roles.

Methods used

This study used an AR approach and provided useful details of data analysis using thematic network (sounds useful ... follow up). The team stated that they did not 'need' to follow a number of cycles within the study, as they felt no further changes required modification after the second meeting when the teaching was introduced.

Example 2

Authors: H. Waterman, D. Tillen, R. Dickson and K. de Koning (2001)

Title: Action Research: A Systematic Review and Guidance for Assessment

Source and details: Health Technology Assessment (Monograph 5). London: Department of Health.

Notes

This report provided a good overview of the origins of action research and a detailed definition. The section on assessing quality in action research projects was particularly useful – worth reading before, during, and after the project ...

Many people find the use of index cards a very practical and simple way of keeping track of what they have read but, if a researcher has a good knowledge of technology, they may be able to set up systems using a computer (in Excel, for example) which will do the same as index cards. If they choose to do so, information retrieval can be much quicker. Having said all this, the most effective recording system will be one which is personal and manageable. Researchers may want to take note of the above guidelines and then design their own systems. Sorting out sources of literature into different categories and themes is also helpful.

In recent times we have gained access to software which enables us to manage references efficiently. *Reference Manager* and *EndNote* are software packages which can be used to organize, store, and retrieve references of research literature. These save time when writing up and beyond. Using *EndNote* one can directly download references from online databases. As with all software packages, it can be useful to work with someone who may have used it before or to attend a training course.

Reading and appraising the literature

Creating a table or a template for recording what has been read can save time and energy. Again, the system created must be personal to the user. If action researchers read about action research carried out by other practitioners, they should take note of the following:

- What was the context of their research?
- Who was involved? Was it an individual or a collaborative project? Was there a facilitator?
- Was the choice of using action research as a method justified? Were any models discussed?
- How were the data analysed?
- Were ethical considerations addressed? How?
- What 'actions' took place?
- How were the data gathered, analysed, and validated?
- What were the conclusions? Were they justified using appropriate evidence?
- Was the report accessible? Useful?
- What items may be useful to think about for another action research study?

Reviewing and writing up any reading

At this stage for researchers it is worth revisiting the purpose of reviewing and writing up the literature. They would be doing this in order to find out what other researchers have found out previously about the topic of inquiry, the key ideas generated by others in the field, and the theories developed by them. There is no one way to do this, but here are some guidelines developed by Koshy (2010):

- Researchers should take note of how other researchers who were involved in similar projects – small scale, Master's or doctoral level – wrote up their literature review in published papers, reports, or theses. It is also important they develop a personal style of presentation which suits the context.
- Researchers should start writing a summary of what they have read, starting with an overview of what the research topic is about and organizing the summaries under sub-headings as themes. Under each sub-heading, an account of the research undertaken highlighting its findings should be written up. It is important not to just write a list of who said or found out what, but to review the findings with an accompanying personal, critical commentary. It is useful to highlight (perhaps in different colours) authors with similar views and findings as well as contrasting ones. There is nothing more tedious, in our opinion, for the reader than reading a list of what each author has said with no reflection on the contents or any inter-connecting commentaries.
- Time spent on creating the literature review is well spent, as it not only gives researchers more confidence in carrying out research, it also saves time later when it comes to writing a final report and the subsequent authorship of journal papers.

Creating a personal conceptual map, a visual summary (Creswell, 2009) of what has been read, may also be useful. Maps can be organized in different ways. A research topic could be placed in the centre or at the top and linked with connecting arrows to boxes which can record different themes and sub-themes and the names of authors and dates. This kind of map can help greatly when writing up a literature review.

Again, note that one of the most important purposes of searching for different sources of literature and reviewing them is to help researchers construct a framework for understanding the issues relating to the topic under investigation. This is done most effectively if researchers can tell the coherent story which emerged from their reading.

The reader may find Koshy's (2010) three-stage plan for writing litera-ture reviews, developed with her education students, useful. This plan is as follows:

1 Identify the significant themes that have emerged from any reading. These would have been highlighted by using written summaries and colour-coded sections while gathering and reading the literature.
2 Introduce the ideas by themes rather than by listing different authors' viewpoints. If a researcher writes in sequence what others have said it can become very tedious and disjointed for the reader.
3 Introduce each theme and explain what that particular theme is. Then present the evidence from any reading, both agreements and disagreements between experts. For example, if a researcher is discussing a particular intervention as a means to improve patient care, explaining what the particular theme means in context and putting forward the views of authors and experts on that theme followed by a critical commentary of any final thoughts is highly effective here.

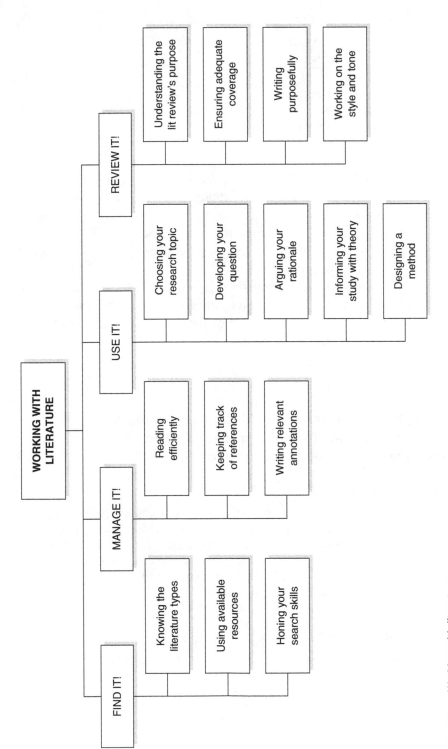

FIGURE 3.1 *Working with literature*

Blaxter et al's (1996: 115) guidance to researchers on writing critical reviews of literature is worthy of consideration. The suggestion is that researchers use references to:

- justify and support the arguments;
- allow comparisons to be made with other research;
- explain matters better than they could have done themselves;
- explain their own familiarity with the field of research.

O'Leary's representation, in Figure 3.1, provides an effective diagrammatic model of how the research process is supported by a literature search and its use. To conclude this chapter, we shall draw on two reported examples of how literature reviews have informed action researchers. We have used the actual publications in order to capture the effectiveness of the contexts and the purposes of the projects.

Example 3.1 reports on a study (Mitchell et al., 2005) undertaken in Northern Ireland which was designed to improve the knowledge and skills of nurses in the moving and handling of patients following a stroke. An extract from the literature review is presented below.

Example 3.1   Towards rehabilitative handling in caring for patients following stroke: a participatory action research project (Mitchell et al., 2005)

Literature review

In action research the purpose of the literature review is not only to ascertain what is already known, but also to generate ideas for changing practice. The CINAHL and MEDLINE databases were searched from 1992–2002. Combinations of the key words of 'stroke', 'manual handling', multidisciplinary care', 'ergonomics' and 'rehabilitation' were used, and citation lists were examined, and articles were identified for review.

Moving and handling practice

In the past decade researchers and educators have called on nurses to scrutinise their moving and handling practice and adhere to Manual Handling Operations regulations. However, there are many studies to indicate that some nurses continue to manually lift using condemned techniques. Gollancz and Thomas (1996) in a national survey (N = 1600) analyzed the written records of

(Continued)

back injured nurses, stored in the Royal College of Nursing's legal departments. Fifty-two percent of these nurses reported injuries sustained in lifting and handling incidents. Some reported that they had continued to use the orthodox lift, although this approach was condemned in 1987. Nurses at junior grade were more likely to sustain injury than more senior nurses and this was interpreted as a consequence of their direct care role.

The Confederation of Health Service Employees (1992) reported that up to 40% of injuries go unreported by nurses. Similarly, Green (1996) found that nurses on two medical wards (N = 10) were reluctant to report injuries sustained in moving and handling incidents. Non-participant observation data identified that risk assessments in relation to moving patients were often incomplete and nurses were continuing to use the orthodox lift. Although this was a small study, qualitative data collection by the use of semi-structured interviews gleaned rich data and Green concluded that nurses had negative attitudes towards changing practice. Training in moving and handling was also deficient as qualified nurses in one ward had received no training in using a hoist (Green, 1996). In a recent Australian survey using a convenient sample of nurses (N = 523) 40% of respondents admitted they were continuing to lift patients manually and were ignoring legislation and practice guidelines (Retsas and Pinikahana, 2000).

(This section continues in the published paper, with all the references included.)

The second project by Grant and Robling (2006) is concerned with the involvement of general practitioners in undergraduate medical practices.

Example 3.2 Introducing undergraduate medical teaching into general practice: an action research study (Grant and Robling, 2006)

The authors state 'we chose an action research approach , which is described as a 'Small scales intervention is the real world' (Cohen et al., 2000). They continue 'Unlike a controlled trial or an observational study, action research involves observation of an intervention, and reflection on its effect, in this case preparation for teaching and teaching itself. The outcomes of the reflection may be to amend the intervention with evaluation by further cycles of action research'. Below is an extract from the article.

The last decade has seen a greater proportion of undergraduate medical education take place in general practice (Society for Academic Primary Care, 2002; Mathers et al., 2004; Morrison and Spencer, 2004). This has largely

(Continued)

(Continued)

been driven by the General Medical Council's report 'Tomorrow's Doctors' (General Medical Council, 1993). In 1996 the number of sessions delivered in general practice in the whole curriculum at British medical schools was between 20 and 40. By 2001 it had increased to an average of 120. In 2002 academic general practice was contributing an average of 9% of the entire undergraduate curriculum (Society for Academic Primary Care, 2002).

Whilst teaching in general practice provides students with enhanced learning opportunities, it requires teaching practices to accommodate more students and more practices to be recruited by medical schools (Mathers et al., 2004)

Community-based education offers a strategy for introducing new health professionals into primary care. In the declaration of Alma Ata (WHO, 1978) it was proposed that teaching health care professionals in the community, away from tertiary care centres, would result in more students, after qualifying, electing to work in primary care with some choosing to go back to the areas where they had trained. The idea was echoed by some general practitioners who, when interviewed, said that students who had enjoyed a good GP placement were more likely to return to the area to practice themselves (Mathers et al., 2004). A number of initiatives have been successful in increasing recruitment of doctors to rural and underserved areas by increasing the proportion of undergraduates teaching those areas (Worly et al., 2000).

(This section continues in the published paper with full references.)

For an action researcher here is a practical task to carry out a literature search and review using some of the ideas we have discussed in this chapter.

Imagine you have been awarded a grant to initiate an action research project to improve an aspect of practice within your institution or work context. First, decide what your area of study is going to be and then carry out a literature search using some of the sources listed in this paper. Search the literature relating to the topic of study as well as finding out if any action research has been carried out on this particular topic. Again, as always, working with a group on this task is much more fun.

Summary

In this chapter we explained the purpose of undertaking literature reviews and have led the reader through the process of searching for relevant literature. Guidance has been given on how to structure the search, evaluate internet sources, and organize the literature. Guidance was provided on the kinds of literature which may be useful for a project. It was also proposed that the fledgling researcher take note of research methods used by other researchers and critically appraise their findings. In this chapter we have attempted to suggest ways in which the action researcher can ease their path through the literature maze.

Further reading

Creswell, J.W. (2009) *Research Design: Qualitative, Quantitative, and Mixed Methods Approaches.* Thousand Oaks, CA: SAGE.

Hart, C. (2001) *Doing a Literature Search: A Comprehensive Guide for the Social Sciences.* London: SAGE/The Open University.

Merriam, S.B. (1998) *Qualitative Research and Case Study Applications in Education.* San Francisco, CA: Jossey-Bass.

O'Dochartaigh, N. (2007) *Internet Research Skills.* London: SAGE.

O'Leary, Z. (2004) *The Essential Guide to Doing Research.* London: SAGE.

4

Steps in the Action Research Process: Practical Considerations

This chapter focuses on:

- The quality of action research projects
- When action research is appropriate
- The stages of action research
- Guidance on planning action research projects
- Examples of action research.

Introduction

The first two chapters of this book focused on general aspects relating to action research: the historical development and distinguishing features of the action research approach were presented in Chapter 1, while the types of inquiry undertaken by healthcare workers and the advantages and the perceived limitations of action research as a methodology were discussed in Chapter 2. Examples of action research projects, carried out in a range of contexts and focusing on a variety of topics provided in previous chapters, show that the underlying common purpose in such practitioner projects is desire to improve their practice within a particular context or situation. An analysis of the reported action research studies demonstrated that the objectives achieved through undertaking the projects could be described under three broad, but inter-related, strands.

First of these is the acquisition of greater powers of critical reflection and self-knowledge acquired by the participants through the action research process, whether a project was initiated by an individual either as part of his or her academic studies, or by groups of healthcare workers working together on a project. Second, in the examples of action research provided in previous chapters, the researchers reported that engaging in action research had encouraged them to develop the skills of team work, professional collegiality, and taking ownership for decisions, as well as feeling a kind of empowerment arising out of their ability to improve and influence aspects of their practice without 'being told' by outside agencies what 'to do'. A third objective achieved by many of the researchers was in terms of the central role played by them in bringing about social change and an enhanced quality of care for the users and quite often this was achieved in situations where power relationships and conflicts posed many challenges. Action researchers' motivation has been a key factor in the success of projects. In this chapter, we shall address some practical issues in carrying out action research, drawing on our own personal experiences and from reading and hearing about action research projects carried out by other researchers.

Quality of action research projects

According to Hughes (2008), the claims that multiple randomized controlled trials are the 'gold standard' of evidence about the value of healthcare interventions are being challenged. Hughes quotes Green (2004) who suggests that if we want more evidence-based practice, we need more practice-based evidence. Although it could be argued that assessing the quality of action research projects should be an 'end' process, we believe it is useful for action researchers to have some awareness of what constitutes a 'good project' at the time of planning and making preparations. This would enable researchers to take a set of quality criteria into account while planning and working on a project. Whilst acknowledging the complexity of establishing a set of quality indictors for action research as a checklist, as 'it would make it difficult to capture the interactions between the different components of action research', Waterman et al. (2001) provide a comprehensive list of 20 questions which may be used to assess action research projects. These guidelines, they suggest, may provide new researchers with a structure on which to develop their work. A summary of the key messages guidance is provided below for consideration, but we would recommend that the reader familiarize themself with the full list of these questions and their associated explanations in the original report. The detailed list provided by Waterman et al. (2001) and based on their systematic review of action research projects encourages action researchers to consider the following issues:

- It is reasonable and useful for researchers and participants to articulate their aims and objectives at the outset, at least for the first phase of the enquiry, although the very nature of action research may make it necessary for sub-objectives to be defined as the project progresses.
- The relevance of the project to local and wider contexts needs to be considered and reported. The project team may consist of healthcare workers from different contexts and the inquiry may result in new understandings within and beyond the immediate situation.
- Some attempts should be made to define the phases of the research. However, it is pointed out that it is difficult to specify, in advance, certain activities or cycles as the outcomes of each phase will inform the next. It is also recommended that the first phase of action research, which includes an initial analysis of the situation under study and which sets the scene for subsequent phases, should be planned and undertaken as thoroughly as possible.
- The appropriate selection and inclusion of participants and stakeholders is described as 'vital' to the success of an action research project. It would be useful to explain how individuals or groups were selected and why their participation was considered important. This includes the role of any outside facilitators. The relationship between researchers and participants should also be thought through and nurtured.
- An understanding of the local context, beliefs, and structures and any possible outcomes and knock-on-effects of the project should be clearly articulated.
- Management issues should be addressed. The roles and responsibilities of the key persons should be established at the outset. The involvement of senior managers and nurses was found to contribute to a greater impact on outcomes.
- Reflexive and ethical considerations need to be addressed (these are discussed in Chapter 5).
- Funding and resource issues need to be planned in advance and any external funding applications should include requests for sufficient funding.
- The time-line and length of the project need to be considered carefully and preparations made in advance. Flexibility should be built into the plans.
- Data collection methods should match the aims and objectives of the project and the plans for data analysis should be rigorous.
- Statements of findings should be clear.
- Some advance thoughts as to the extent to which the aims and objectives would be met should be considered, along with a consideration of whether the findings could be transferable.
- The researchers should consider and report the criteria on which their work is to be read and judged.

The following set of general questions for assessing the quality of action research projects, are based on advice from Bradbury and Reason (2002).

Action researchers must ensure that:

- they acknowledge their world views.
- all members of the group are actively involved.
- the research is conceptually sound.
- they select appropriate methods.
- the research gives practical and theoretical knowledge.
- their work leads to better understanding and change of practice.

Time for action: rhetoric into practice

A review of published studies in healthcare related journals and websites shows that there is a gradual increase in the use of the action research approach, either in the context of responding to new national initiatives or for localized improvements to services. There is also greater involvement by user groups in projects designed to improve the quality of healthcare, though more of this would be desirable. Recent developments in the UK have witnessed a number of national initiatives which have recommended approaches that are consistent with the features of action research. For example, the current UK government's desire to 'decentralize' and 'encourage local decision making' and 'community involvement' is expressed clearly in the context of the setting up of Foundation Trusts (NHS, 2005). The call for introducing 'innovative' and 'flexible' approaches to healthcare opens up many possibilities for adopting an action research approach within healthcare settings as it provides a methodology for implementing change, where a group of researchers is willing to work together on identifying issues and improving practice.

What is perhaps required to turn rhetoric into practice is a cultural shift in terms of more rewards and a greater acknowledgement of research in localized and applied contexts. The establishment of reflective and developmental projects that are necessary to be successful in action research may be challenging, as traditional incentives often reward quantitative predicable research. As Feldman (2008) points out, another related hurdle is that journal publication norms often require the tight control of experimental conditions and these are difficult to achieve in real-world contexts.

Other recent developments in the UK which have encouraged more *applied research* that can lead to greater user involvement and a faster impact on healthcare have been recommended by CLAHRC (Collaboration for

Leadership in Applied Health Research and Care) and supported by the National Institute for Health Research (NIHR). An example of the CLAHRC initiative (there are nine altogether) can be seen in the vision statement of the Northwest London group, hosted by the Chelsea and Westminster Hospital NHS Foundation Trust in partnership with Imperial College, London. While writing this chapter an action research workshop was being offered as part of the support activities of this group. Several elements of the vision statement of the group, outlined below, show the potential for action research projects. These state that the vision is to continuously improve the quality of patient care by accelerating the implementation of evidence-based research and innovations into practice and that it will do this by:

- engaging patients and the public in having a voice in the design and delivery of new innovations and improvements;
- fostering a culture of change across northwest London through the development of a continuous improvement capacity and the increased implementation of evidence-based research;
- supporting and empowering the local health system through the provision of training and development;
- developing and evaluating systematic implementation processes to expedite the delivery of evidence-based research to patients.

Service user engagement is a key component of all NIHR CLAHRC services across the UK. We can see clearly how the key principles enabled within an action research approach, such as participation, collaboration, researching in localized contexts, improvement, empowerment, and user engagement could be applied within these initiatives.

The third author is involved in part of the Greater Manchester CLAHRC which is a collaboration between 19 NHS primary and Secondary Care Trusts in Greater Manchester and the University of Manchester. In this CLAHRC, a series of inter-related interventions to support patient self-management and improve the quality of care for people with chronic vascular disease will be researched. Some of these projects will use action research and involve users in the process. Additionally, several projects aim to implement existing research to improve the care of those with long-term vascular conditions. In the implementation strand, action research will be employed as a methodology to understand the facilitation of knowledge utilization by staff. This project involves six people whose responsibility it is to facilitate the implementation of research to improve patient care across eight different projects. They will be working as co-researchers in a co-learning and co-researching process.

During some work relating to the Qualities and Outcomes Framework (QOF) for general practices in England, Wales, and Scotland, the first author of this book identified the potential for a number of action research projects. QOF offers a system for resourcing and rewarding general practitioners (GPs) within the National Health Service in England (http://www.qof.ic.hhs.uk/). The QOF has undergone some changes since it was introduced in 2004; the latest set of indicators or measures of achievement for general practices are based on:

- clinical care, with indicators across 19 clinical areas (such as coronary heart disease, hypertension);
- organizational, with 36 indicators across five organizational areas (such as records and information, information for patients, education and training);
- patient experiences, with five indicators that relate to length of consultation and patient care;
- additional services, with eight indicators across four services (such as child health surveillances, cervical screening).

The potential for setting up action research projects relating to most areas of QOF, within single practices or across practices in a geographical area, is clear. As action research studies within general practices are smaller in number compared to other healthcare settings, there are many potential opportunities that can be identified. One specific example of this would be to set up studies to explore situations relating to *exception reporting* by general practices, so as not to lose credit points on account of circumstances which may be beyond their control. This refers to the possibility afforded to general practices to exclude patients from performance reporting for reasons such as drug intolerance or patient refusal (Koshy, 2008). It is allowed for a number of cases, but it has been reported that younger people and those from lower socio-economic backgrounds are often in this category. Studies designed to explore the reasons for this and to develop strategies to achieve greater equity and social justice are thus worthy of consideration.

In the context of general practice, one question that the first author has been asked during the initial discussions about writing this book and since by her colleagues is: 'What is the difference between the usual audits carried out by general practices and action research?' The main difference is that action research involves the systematic collection of a range of data, analysis, evaluation, and critical reflection on both the process and outcomes of the project (Waterman, 1996). Another is that the evidence is rigorously monitored and disseminated at some level with the potential to generate and add to existing knowledge on a specific issue. In all such initiatives, what is needed is more encouragement and support – in terms of more training and opportunities for practitioner-initiated projects in local contexts.

When is action research appropriate?

In order to address this question, let us remind ourselves of some of the salient features of action research. Lingard et al. (2008) state that the key features of action research include its collaborative nature, its egalitarian approach to power and education in the research process, and taking action on an issue. They also stress that the extensive collaboration between researchers and partners in action research must extend across each stage of the research, from identifying the problem to disseminating the results. In Table 4.1 we list some possible contexts which are suitable for action research and consider when action research may not be an appropriate approach.

Contexts for action research

The examples of action research projects presented in this book show that they were set in a variety of contexts and addressed a range of issues. In

TABLE 4.1   *Contexts in which action research is or is not appropriate*

When it is appropriate to carry out action research	When it may not be appropriate to carry out action research
An action research approach is suitable:	An action research approach may not be suitable:
• when the participants are motivated by a common desire to improve an existing situation, or solve a problem in a local context	• when the intention is to conduct experiments in the use of a new or existing drug or line of treatment
• when trying to develop ways of implementing a new policy effectively	• when there are too many competing priorities within the institution, and time and energy cannot be spared
• when exploring how best to apply the findings of an experimental study in a practical context	• when there is resistance to change within the institution
• when a group of colleagues feel there is a need for change in the level of existing services or in the quality of what is offered	• when significant changes of staff are expected
• when seeking effective ways to implement clinical guidelines	• when there is a lack of resources
• when participants feel that an intervention may have the potential to create more efficient organizational structures within an institution	• when there is a policy which is enforced externally and cannot be changed locally
• when there are support structures in place, through funding from local authorities for implementing change or when an external facilitator suggests a useful idea or innovation	• when it is to be used to study and/or assess the clinical competencies of workers

their analysis of 47 action research projects, Waterman et al. (2001) listed the main issues addressed by the projects as:

- Professional education and skills training (14), which included issues relating to deficits in and the potential for professional development and, more specifically, the usefulness of educational strategies and their delivery.
- Issues relating to inappropriate educational approaches which were of concern in some studies that included professional profiles, clinical supervision, and core nursing skills.
- Issues relating to inappropriate or conflicting practices (13) which were of concern in some studies which included clinical care and policy and educational interventions.
- Studies which addressed a lack of evidence (12) to support existing approaches and innovations which were in areas of organizational change and development.
- Studies looking at professional roles (10) which were concerned with the clarification and development of new and existing roles as well as exploring the barriers to their uptake.
- Other contexts for research included health service provision, communication and/or involvement, targets and guidelines, the implementation of research in practice, and power-related topics.

As a practical task for the reader we have presented examples of some studies below which have been adapted from abstracts and the summaries of published research projects (any direct mention of the research approach has been deliberately removed from them). Only some of these studies were carried out as action research projects. Based on the discussions in previous sections of this book on action research and its features, try to identify which of these were carried out as action research. Think of the reasons why you have made a particular decision. Working with a partner or group should generate useful discussions. Only after doing this, read on to see if you were right in your decisions. Full titles and references for the examples are given at the end of the book.

Study 1: Esprit study group (Halker et al., 2006)

This study reported on the results of trials of aspirin and dipyridamole combined versus aspirin alone for the secondary prevention of vascular events after an ischaemic stroke of presumed arterial origin which were inconsistent. The aim of the research was to resolve this uncertainty. The results showed that this study, combined with the results of previous trials, provided sufficient evidence to prefer the combination regimen of aspirin plus dipyridamole over aspirin alone as antithrombotic therapy after cerebral ischaemia of arterial origin.

Study 2: Mitchell et al., 2005

The objectives of this study were to: facilitate nurses in sharing their insights in moving and handling patients following a stroke, enable nurses to identify the facilitators of safer moving and handling practices, empower nurses in collaboration with physiotherapists to direct changes in their practice.

Study 3: Koshy et al., 2008

This study was set up to investigate the effectiveness of using Short Message Service (SMS) appointment reminders as a cost effective and time-efficient strategy to decrease non-attendance and so improve the efficiency of out-patient healthcare delivery in a hospital Ophthalmology department. The study used a control group.

Study 4: Hassett et al., 2003

The background to this study was that few data exist concerning the natural history of lumbar spine disc degeneration and its associated risk factors. Therefore the authors undertook this study in order to examine the radiographic progression of lumbar spine disc degeneration over the course of nine years in a population-based inception cohort of women from the Chingford Study. The authors demonstrated progression rates of 3–4% per annum, with important risk factors for progression, including age, back pain, and radiographic OA at the hip and knee.

Study 5: Leighton, 2005

This project involved studying the experiences of people in one mental health rehabilitation unit where a conventional individualized approach had repeatedly failed. The research was used to identify the key problems concerned, construct appropriate goals, and formulate problem-solving plans.

Study 6: Reed, 2005

This study reports research which was developed following the findings of a previous inquiry, which had indicated that older people moving from hospital to care homes were not given opportunities to discuss their concerns and preferences with hospital staff. It proposed to develop and implement a 'Daily Living Plan' which was aimed to specify lifestyle preferences. Staff from six wards and seven staff from care homes were involved in the project, which reported some successful outcomes, but the project also highlighted some problems relating to shared ownership of the project.

Study 7: Kelly et al., 2002

This project was set up to evaluate the clinical practice facilitator role for junior nurses in an acute hospital setting. The objectives of the project were: to pilot and evaluate the role of the Clinical Practice Facilitator (CPF), to determine the key factors which contributed to the success of such posts, and to develop a framework for CPF practice to support its function and to identify the future potential of the role in the trust. The project was carried out in three phases: assessment, action, and evaluation.

Study 8: Dolan et al., 2004

The background to this study was that the availability of access to bone densitometry in the UK varies widely and there are concerns as to appropriate prescribing. Studies suggest the inadequate use of osteoporosis prophylaxis in steroid users, despite recent guidelines. The objective was to examine whether access to bone densitometry affected GPs' osteoporosis prescribing in high-risk steroid users. It was found that GPs were three times more likely to start potent osteoporosis treatment after abnormal scans than GPs relying on clinical information. In practice, risk factors were not adequately assessed. Database searches may identify patients needing osteoporosis prophylaxis; however, DXA enables more appropriate patient treatment.

Study 9: Kumar et al., 2009

The objective of this study was to understand why GPs prescribed antibiotics for some cases of a sore throat and to explore the factors that influenced their prescribing. The setting was general practice involving 40 general practitioners (25 in the maximum variety sample and 15 in the theoretical sample). Results showed that general practitioners were uncertain about which patients would benefit from antibiotics but prescribed for sicker patients and for those who came from socio-economically deprived backgrounds because of concerns about complications. They were also more likely to prescribe in pressured clinical contexts. Doctors were mostly comfortable with their prescribing decisions and were not prescribing to maintain the doctor-patient relationship.

Study 10: Lindsey and McGuinness, 1998

The research question guiding this study was aimed at identifying the significant elements of community involvement. A research approach was used in order to address issues of research relevance, community involvement, democracy, emancipation, and liberation. Five themes emerged from the project; (a) planning for participation; (b) the structural component of community participation; (c) living the philosophy; (d) enhancing the credibility; and (e) the type of leadership required to facilitate community participation.

Below the reader can find out if they had identified the studies which used an action research approach.

1   This study was conducted as a randomized controlled trial.
2   This was conducted as a participatory action research project.
3   This was an observational study.
4   This was a first population based, longitudinal study.
5   This study used an action research approach.
6   This was carried out using an action research approach.
7   This was an action research study.
8   This was a case–control study.
9   This qualitative study used a Grounded Theory approach.
10 This was an action research study.

Stages in carrying out action research

In this section we shall discuss the practical aspects of setting up and carrying out an action research project. Whilst acknowledging that action research offers a unique paradigm of inherent flexibility, we feel it would be useful to consider the different stages in some kind of sequence from the outset. Such a list can be useful to both facilitators and participants for the purpose of planning and preparation. Although the models of action research from experts, presented in earlier chapters, suggest that action research is cyclical in nature with distinct stages of setting up the project (planning, acting, observing, evaluating, and reflecting) in reality these stages are often inter-linked and will overlap. We would also like to point out that reflection, which is a key component of the action research process, should ideally feature at each stage. So, for action researchers who are about to start a project, thinking about the following stages may help to gain some insight into what to expect.

The stages may be described as:

- identifying a topic;
- reflection;
- reviewing and analysing the literature;
- focusing on a topic or issue or formulating a research question;
- planning activities;
- implementing and acting;
- gathering and analysing data;
- evaluating;
- reflecting on the outcomes and generating evidence;
- repeating the cycle;
- reporting on the findings.

Rather than discussing each of the stages separately, we will do this using four phases:

1   Identification of an issue and setting up a project.
2   Reflection.
3   The planning stage.
4   The evaluation stage.

Identification of an issue and setting up a project

During this stage, the participants will discuss and identify a specific concern, issue, or problem to solve. This would be something identified by researchers as desirable to change and worthwhile for their efforts. An introductory literature review, discussion, and reflection should help to decide on suitable fruitful directions to explore and on how to proceed. It is possible that the project may be in response to a new policy initiative and seeking the most effective ways of implementing it, or it may be that the researchers will be considering if an intervention, which has worked in a similar setting to theirs, can be implemented.

Some practical questions for researchers to consider at this stage are:

- What is the problem or issue we need to work on?
- What is the justification for investing our time and effort?
- Thinking ahead, what would be the outcomes of the project?
- What might the changed situation look like (this can either be pre-determined or arise as a result of the project)?

During this stage, the following aspects of participation also need to be considered:

- Who will be involved in the project? Are they sufficiently interested?
- Is there a project leader or facilitator?
- Will it involve a multi-disciplinary team?
- What would be the management structure?
- How should issues of power be considered?
- Will the stakeholders and users be involved?

General practical issues to consider at this stage

Motivation and interest

A topic or research question for an action research enquiry will be located within a researcher's experience and context. It needs to be grounded in the realities of the workplace. A researcher needs to ask if they are sufficiently interested in the topic of investigation to devote a considerable amount of their time and effort to it. In our experience, personal interest and commitment are important factors which motivate all researchers and this is the same for an action researcher. Many of the examples we have included in this book bear testimony to the benefits of undertaking action researcher projects, as described by the researchers themselves, at both personal and professional levels. In most cases, the impact of their efforts on the institutions involved has been considerable.

The research topic or question

If the action research involves investigating a question, a researcher needs to consider the type of question which is appropriate to ask. A consideration of the expected outcomes may help in phrasing this question. A researcher will need to consider whether the question should be specific or open-ended in nature. They may wish to explore a specific question with the possibility of multiple outcomes. What they hope to achieve will remain tentative and speculative at the start, as they will be making conjectures about the outcomes. Whether the issue a researcher wishes to investigate is based on an intuitive insight, or arising from their curiosity, they will need to be open-minded in their collection and analysis of the data.

Scope and resources

Action research projects should have a clear focus and they are quite often small-scale investigations. A researcher needs to select topics which are manageable. The aim of an action research inquiry is not to change the world but to bring about an improvement in practice or to implement some changes within an institution. Of course, by sharing findings and dissemination activities, other researchers will read or hear about a project and may wish to transfer these to their study. A researcher must ask what they can possibly achieve in the time-scale available to them and be realistic. They also need to consider the external factors that may affect the project. For example, do they have enough resources to carry out the project? Considering this question in terms of the availability of time, people, and physical material is vital. Do they, for example, have support for word processing and transcribing tapes? A researcher must consider if the participants are likely to change their responsibilities or move on during the scheduled time of the project, or if the institution intends to embark on another initiative at the same time. These issues may be fatal for a project, so it is important for a researcher to anticipate and minimize any problems.

Planning

The importance of planning cannot be over-emphasized. Aims must be made clear and objectives must be listed unambiguously. If there is an action research group, researchers will do this together and plan activities which relate to the achievement of the objectives. Researchers must spend time considering the kind of data they will need to collect and the processes involved in data collection. It is also important they think about how they may analyse and validate the data. It is useful here to initiate a literature search as soon as they have a selected a topic for consideration and to start making notes and summaries. In light of what researchers read, it may be necessary for them to refine or even change the direction of the topic.

Working collaboratively

An important feature of action research is that it offers opportunities for collaborative work. As the old saying goes, 'many hands make light work' and this also increases feelings of ownership and a willingness to change practice. The need for collaboration and co-operation is of paramount importance for the success of a project. A researcher may be part of a group of action researchers. Whether they are leading the project or contributing to it, teamwork is essential here. If a researcher is in a leadership role, it is important they show that they value everyone's contributions. If they are a co-researcher it is necessary for them to listen and share perspectives as often as they can possibly manage it. But they must also remember that it is not always easy to accept critical comments on something that people have spent hours preparing or doing. The need to establish trust and respect for colleagues is, therefore, paramount. To help smooth the process of collaboration especially within the action research group, it is vital researchers discuss and agree on the ground rules for behaviour in meetings. For example, they might want to agree that no-one will be ridiculed and that the meetings should be constructive.

Consider dissemination

Finally, a researcher must consider the question of: what will they do with the findings when the project is complete? It is important, from the start, that they give some thought to how the project findings will be disseminated. If they need to send a report to a funding body, there may be a specific format to follow. Are they intending perhaps to make a conference presentation or lead a professional development course? Would they consider writing for a professional journal? They may be doing this project as part of studies at a university leading to a dissertation. In all these cases, it will be useful to look to the future and think about the final stages of the project.

Reflection

Reflection in the context of action research

Group and individual reflection is crucial to action research. We view it as the glue that binds the other components of action and research together. Reflection is not normally a feature of conventional quantitative research. In qualitative research, personal researcher reflections are noted down in diaries but they are not usually shared or critiqued within a group of co-researchers. Reflective practice is common in healthcare practice and has many similarities to reflection in action research. These are: that it is carried out in groups over a specified time period; that participants identify the problem aspects of practice; that they review that practice and support one another to find constructive ways forward. However, participants will normally work on individual professional issues and that means the group will examine several different problems, whereas in action research any reflection is aimed at examining and resolving one group problem. Another difference between reflective practice and reflection in action research is that the latter is part of a research project leading to new knowledge that may be published. Reflection in action research runs alongside all the stages of action research and feeds into these and conversely the outcomes from all these stages may feed into reflective meetings. The person who has set up the action research may be best situated to be the moderator (facilitator) of the reflection initially and then as the group proceeds participants might wish to take turns at moderating. Note that most participants will need training and practice before taking on this role.

Frameworks for reflection

Frameworks for reflection in action research are useful to structure meetings but, on the other hand, they might inhibit the free flow of discussion.

The action research group should decide on whether they should use a framework and if so which one, checking that it fits with the aspirations of the project. We have adapted Kemmis and McTaggart's (1988) detailed set of questions to assist with the reflective process.

- Language

    - *What are the key ideas relating to what needs to change?*
      For example, in an action research project to promote face down posturing after retinal surgery, it was realized that patients were described as 'not doing as they were told'. This discourse revealed that practitioners had an authoritative relationship with patients and were not working with them to improve the situation. It can be very revealing to examine the commonly used language regarding the issue under study as it can show taken-for-granted values.

    - *What is the history of current explanations for a behaviour?*
      For example, it was the tradition to tell patients to lie face down for several weeks after surgery after recovering from the anaesthetic. The pre-operative clinics where patients could have been told about the need for posturing were perceived by staff to be far too busy to accommodate any more patients. There was an assumption that this was the only way to behave.

    - *What policies exist and whose interests do they serve?*
      For example, each consultant had a slightly different policy for how many minutes in each hour the patient should posture, ranging from 45 minutes out of each 60-minute span to no relief at all. These policies aimed to safeguard the interests of patients but there was no evidence to support which was best.

    - *What contestations exist over language?*
      For example, patients tended to blame staff for the lack of clear timely instructions, while nurses blamed the doctors for not giving clear instructions and doctors often blamed the nurses for not getting the patients into position. This meant that each group was blaming everybody but themselves for the situation.

    - *Does the language reflect what actually happens in practice?*
      For example, the rhetoric of individualized patient care contradicted the actual care received by some patients. This meant that staff were not behaving according to their espoused professional values.

- Relevant activities and practice

    - *What activities are patients and staff involved in with regard to the problem?*
      This could be studied through observation of a practice or by following patients as they pass through the system. For example, we observed the nursing care of patients immediately after surgery as they learnt to posture face down. By doing this, we also learnt that the standard of care was variable but saw examples of excellent nursing care that could be the basis for future staff training.

    - *What role do patients and each professional play? Do they have control over their own roles?*
      For example, we learnt that it was the doctors' role to clearly communicate the post-operative instructions to patients and ward staff, it was the nurses' role to

be educators and advocate for patients, and it was the patients' role to ask questions if they did not understand what was expected of them.

o   *Are there viable alternatives to the way everyone acts now?*
     For example, if the clinic structure was reviewed could a slot for a pre-operative clinic for these patients be found so that they could receive information about posturing before the day of surgery? In addition, could patients be given clear readable pictures of the posture that was required rather than just oral instructions?

- Social relationships and the organization

  o   *What are the key organizational structures and social relationships which create or constrain opportunities regarding the area of concern?*
       For example, the doctors had a clinic two days a week and the rest of the clinic slots were taken up by other consultants. Traditionally, doctors and nurses had provided scant advice about posturing at the clinic appointment. A nurse specialist was thought to be key in creating opportunities for patient education.

  o   *What relationships of collaboration, cooperation, consultation, control, and coercion exist?*
       For example, there was little collaboration between medical and nursing staff until a nurse specialist was appointed who could liaise between the different groups. Patients were provided with little control over posturing as the instructions were given too late. They were then coerced into complying with them.

  o   *How could these structures and relationships be improved for the benefit of all, especially the patient?*
       For example, patients could have been given control by having such information provided at a pre-operative clinic in advance of the surgery and the communication between nurses and medical staff could have been given greater priority via the appointment of a nurse specialist.

The outcome of the first series of group reflections would be a better understanding of the problem, an identification of those areas requiring further investigation, and a suggestion of any ideas and a desire for change.

Example of group reflection

One of our PhD students from Nigeria carried out a reflection with a village community as part of an action research project to improve maternal mortality. The action research group consisted of women of childbearing age, a male and female community leader, a clergyman, two mothers-in-law, two medical doctors, a traditional birth attendant, a representative of the Director of Nursing Services, and the PhD student herself. This group was selected as it represented the key stakeholders in the birthing process. This group met on four occasions to reflect on maternal mortality. The aims of the reflection were to discuss critically the perceived causes of maternal mortality in the community and from that to identify any possible interventions that would help to prevent maternal mortality.

The reader will have begun to realize by now that action researchers need to have excellent interpersonal as well as research skills in order to be successful.

The planning stage

Researchers need to have selected a topic for research and reflected on the different aspects of that topic. With an enhanced level of understanding of issues, acquired through reading, discussing and reflecting, they will have sharpened their focus and formulated a research question. The next stage is to plan the activities which may take different forms depending on the nature of the project. Researchers may be planning an intervention, designing a model of innovative practice, or developing a new educational strategy. The action may involve a series of changes in existing practices, based on practical considerations or in the light of new evidence or clinical guidelines. Other activities may target improvements in the quality of patient care, the provision of clearer information to users, or the improvement of organizational structures. Or this may involve taking a closer look at professional roles and the career development of the people involved.

A common purpose of all planned activities is to influence practice and often to bring about change in an existing situation. All participants should ideally be involved in the planning process. A more extensive literature search and review may be useful at this stage. Decisions about what kind of data – qualitative, quantitative, or a mixture of both – and how to gather these will have to be made. All the participants will be included in the collection and analysis of data and in making sense of the emerging themes and findings. Researchers' own observations and interpretations of the findings will be shared with the participants during this stage to monitor both the processes and outcomes. It is important that during this time of practical activity, on-going discussion and reflection continue as the evidence of effectiveness is generated. Practical activities at this stage would include seeking ethical clearance and securing permission from the Trust to carry out the research. A project information sheet must be circulated to the relevant people. Establishing a time-line and a list of the resources required will also help to make the project run smoothly.

Action researchers may consider drawing up a conceptual map of their project at this stage. This could be carried out as a shared activity with all those involved in the project – with the research question or issue at the centre and branches outlining the different lines of enquiry, data-gathering methods, and any details about the roles and responsibilities of various participants. More formally a research proposal will need to be written and sent for external peer review and any feedback returned before submission to the ethics committee. If this is something new researchers should seek the assistance of someone who can advise on this. The questions below can act as a guide.

- Do all the participants understand what is involved and the level of commitment required?
- Are any research tools and training required?
- What data will be collected?
- Will the data-gathering methods generate what is required to achieve the objectives of the project?
- How will the data be processed and analysed?
- Have meetings been set up to discuss the findings and ways forward? How often will they take place?
- How will the findings be validated?
- What resources are required? Books, journals, hardware, software, tapes for recording, people to assist with transcribing or analysing data?
- How will any ethical issues be addressed?

Other more general practical questions would include asking:

- Is the project timing suitable? (The answer would probably be 'no' if there are other priorities to deal with or a major change of staff is expected.)
- Is the project manageable?
- Is it ethical?
- Is it methodologically rigorous?
- Is the time plan realistic?
- Will an external facilitator be involved?
- Have power relationships been considered and how may these affect the running of the project?

An action research planning sheet

Completing a planning sheet may be a helpful exercise at the start of a project. This can be discussed with the action research group, before completing it. We have included a commentary here, but a blank grid should be completed for a specific project.

- Our topic of inquiry is about …

- Why do we wish to research this topic?

- *At this stage, a researcher may only have a general idea about the area of study but should write down all relevant ideas.*
- *There could be different reasons for this. Reading or hearing something about the topic, or professional reasons such as a*

new responsibility within an institution or attending a professional conference. Or perhaps because that institution needs to fulfil the requirements of a new health policy. Or perhaps it may be that an institution has applied for funding to undertake an action research project on realizing that an improvement/change to practice is required.

- What is the working title?
- *This may take several attempts. From all the ideas, the most elegant and focused title which conveys the intentions clearly should be selected.*

- What is the research question or aspect that is the study's focus?

- What is known about this?
- *Any initial knowledge about the topic can be recorded here. What readings and literature are available? A conceptual map may help. Include any relevant policy here.*

- Where will the search for literature be focused?
- *Chapter 3 should give plenty of guidance on this.*
- Who will be involved in the research?
- *This requires a list of those people who will be involved and in what capacity. How can their participation be encouraged?*

- What ethical procedures should be put in place?
- *This needs a brief statement about what arrangements need to be made for ethical clearance.*

- What is the time-line?
- *This requires the next meeting date for the ethics committee. A realistic time-line must then be constructed showing the different anticipated phases of the project.*

- What kind of data should be collected? Why are these needed?
- *This requires a list of the kinds of data needed and next to it a justification on why these are necessary and the methods researchers intend to use.*

- Are the plans workable?
- *This needs a list of the possible challenges. Perhaps a lack of time? Colleagues may not hold the same views and may even block the progress of the project. Researchers need to anticipate this and make a list of these challenges.*

- Having completed the grid so far, does anything need to change in the plan? A list is necessary record the reasons.

This is an important stage in all
research activities.

- What are the possible outcomes of
  the research?

- *Researchers should list the possible
  benefits and outcomes, both personal and
  professional, for the people they work
  with and for the institution. They may
  also need to think about any knowledge
  that may be generated that could be
  shared with others.*

- What is the final choice of topic or
  research question?

- *This may have changed after the
  completion of previous sections of this
  grid and if not this section will still
  require researcher attention. Good luck
  with the project!*

The evaluation stage

In an action research project the end point will not always be clearly
marked. The project may come to an end according to the time-scale, but
it is likely that learning and some activities will continue. So what we discuss here is based on assuming that the project ends according to the
planned time-scale of the project. At this stage, the group will be evaluating
the project in terms of the implementation of the activities that were
planned. These may include an intervention, the introduction of new strategies, or an assessment of the existing structures or a consideration of
professional roles. Interviews with users, stakeholders, and managers, may
have to take place and evidence from all the sources about the impact of
the research will need to be included in a final report. A researcher must
be cautious about any claims they make about the effect of an intervention
from having carried out a before and after experimental design. One useful format for carrying out an evaluation of outcomes – both processes and
any products – could be through a reflective discussion, which could be
recorded using a pre-designed evaluation form of the following questions.
A researcher could ask:

- What is the impact of the research for me as a person?
- Has the group benefited? And if so, in what way?
- What is the impact of the project on our institution? Has anything changed from
  what was happening before?
- What knowledge has been generated?
- What are the major lessons learnt?
- If we were doing something similar again, would we change anything ?

- What are the limitations of the project?
- What are the implications for practitioners?

An interesting response to the first question, about personal benefits from a health worker (Charlotte) based in a hospital, included the following.

- Enhanced confidence.
- Greater awareness of my role as a midwife.
- The ability to reflect and be self-critical.
- Greater empowerment.

Waterman et al's quotation from a member of a focus group on the experience of being an action researcher illuminates similar sentiments:

> I think the exciting thing about this whole business of research is that it stimulates people to be self critical, to ask questions, to analyze what they are doing, to check out better ways of doing things. It just stimulates this whole process of enquiry – asking questions, helping people – so they themselves take things forward. I think this is a healthy productive way to operate. (2001: 25)

What are the qualities of an effective action researcher?

When planning action research projects, it is also useful to consider the desirable qualities of an action researcher. So what are these? If the reader belongs to an action research group it might be helpful to discuss this in the group. Below we have listed the qualities one may have already or those that are desirable to develop.

The action researcher:

- needs to be motivated and to stay motivated, and also needs to be able to motivate other people who are working on a project;
- should have a high degree of interpersonal skills and the ability to work in a team;
- should be able to be self-critical, to accept constructive criticism, and to be open-minded;
- should be open to innovative ideas;
- should have the capacity to engage in analysis;
- should have the ability to communicate, both verbally and when reporting in an accessible style;
- should be willing to be challenged;
- should believe that theory and practice can be developed side by side;
- should be flexible and able to respond to unexpected problems and hurdles;
- should be able to work in a collaborative situation, accept any tensions, and try to resolve them.

These bullet points highlight the challenging nature of action research. We can recall students lamenting that they wished they had carried out a survey as this would have been easier than trying to implement and study change. Certainly action research is not an easy option but when successful it can be very rewarding.

When things go wrong

As is the case with most plans we make in everyday life, even after thorough planning and making an effort, things can go wrong at any stage of research. To highlight just a few of these: participants may leave during the project; ethics clearance may take longer than expected; funds and resources may be insufficient to complete the project. Colleague absences can also create problems, especially if the research involves a very small group. And action plans and data collection may not always go according to plan. Or the peer reviewer may suggest that the data collection methods are flawed and the project may have to start all over again, which could challenge the validity of the findings. Some problems that might arise may be due to conflicts with colleagues and power relationships. A researcher needs to anticipate these and various conversations need to take place prior to the start of the project. Reading as many examples of other action research projects and talking to experienced action researchers is valuable here. Many organizational and resource related problems can be avoided if these can be anticipated during the planning stage. For example, when we started out as action researchers we can remember being advised to carry out observation as it would offer the sort of insight that no other method could provide. We decided to follow this advice and found it to be extremely helpful in understanding the context of the problems we were experiencing.

Practical examples of the process of action research

To conclude this chapter, we would invite the reader to engage in a practical task beginning with having a look at the following two summaries of examples of action research projects. They are invited to make a note of the process of action research (especially the planning phase) aimed at encouraging them to reflect on the principles and processes involved in carrying out action research in Chapters 1 and 2. To make it more fun, the reader should imagine they have been awarded a grant of £20,000 to initiate a project to improve an aspect of practice in their work context. The reader may wish to set up a community of researchers with an inter-disciplinary team or with neighbouring institutions. They should make a detailed plan of how they would carry out the project. The reader should not forget to include a breakdown of the expenses they will need to meet. Note that this is an ideal group activity. The examples are different in their settings, scope and their professional contexts and are presented in detail (especially the first of these, which was carried out in the UK). We would highly recommend that the reader access the actual papers (in their entirety) to capture the essence of their contents. Full details are given in the reference section of this book.

Example 4.1   The Keele community knee pain forum: action research to engage with stakeholders about the prevention of knee pain and disability (Jinks et al., 2009)

The authors describe an action research project which involved users in healthcare research.

Background

The aim of this study was to establish a community knee pain forum which engaged stakeholders in the design, dissemination, and prioritization of knee pain research. The study highlighted the benefits, strengths, and challenges in involving users in healthcare. The researchers used INVOLVE (http://www.invo.org.uk/) as a model for the involvement of members in the forum (consultation, collaboration, and user control), which included nine stages: for example, identifying and prioritizing the topics for research and designing, managing, commissioning, undertaking, and disseminating practice. The authors followed the definition of INVOLVE as being based on the need for 'an active partnership between consumers and researchers in the research process, rather than the use of consumers as the subjects of research' (Buckland et al., 2007). They outlined their rationale for the user involvement, as patients often had insights and expertise that complemented those of the healthcare professionals and their involvement in the research may thus improve its quality and impact, legitimacy and value, as well as the identification of gaps to improve the uptake of the research findings.

This externally-funded project, known as KNEPP (Knee Prevention Project), involved users in various stages of the research which consisted of three

(Continued)

(Continued)

linked parts: a systematic review of the risk factors for the onset and progression of knee pain in the community; a National Health Service record review to assess any inequalities in access to healthcare for knee pain in older adults; and a qualitative study to identify perceptions of knee pain prevention in adults of 50 years old or over and in people who worked with older people with knee pain. The users were drawn from a broad spectrum – patients with knee pain and people who would ultimately use the results of the research for patient benefit (for example, local health or community group workers). Ethical approval was obtained from the Local Research Ethics Committee.

Action phase

The first task was to set up the context for the group to operate. The preparatory phase involved identifying the stakeholders, informing them of the study, and gaining their consent to participate. A snowballing technique was used to identify potential forum members, initially by using local knowledge from health services and voluntary and community organizations. The researchers wrote to people explaining the study and the role that the forum had within the study. Ten people were recruited to the forum representing a wide range of agencies, which included Weight Watchers, the leisure industry, charitable agencies and health and social care professionals, and the public. Three university researchers were also involved. There were no expectations that the different stakeholders had different roles in the forum. The aim was to bring together a mixed group which could share a common interest in using the results of the research. Three two-hour meetings, over a two-year period, were held at key points. Each meeting had clear objectives and at the end these were revisited and the main conclusions were agreed upon. The meetings were facilitated by two of the authors who had had previous experience of qualitative interviewing and running focus groups. The team was cognizant of the need to ensure that lay members did not feel overwhelmed by professionals as this was a possibility in a mixed group. Support was given in between meetings so that lay members could contribute fully.

A short evaluation form was mailed to all members after each meeting asking for feedback on the key issues discussed. The final evaluations contained open questions and asked about expectations and experiences of involvement and what should be done differently in the future. At the last meeting, summary conclusions from the forum were debated focusing on key findings, dissemination, and questions for further research. Detailed notes were taken at all meetings backed up by tape recordings. The themes for analysis were separated into processes at the forum and any outcomes that affected the KNEPP study as a whole.

Qualitative interviews were undertaken with people about their understanding of the prevention of knee pain and disability in older adults and what the key determinants were.

During the first meeting with members of the forum, advice was gained on potential methods for the study. A summary of the key tasks and characteristics of each task was included. An established model of heath determinants, developed by Dahlgren and Whitehead (1993), was discussed which the participants commented on and suggested adaptations and additions. Fruitful discussions occurred during meetings on the development of dissemination strategies and the identification of research priorities. Patients were interviewed by recruiting those who had agreed to take part in previous research. General practitioners, doctors and health workers were also interviewed. The university facilitators undertook the systematic review, the presentation of the on-going results, and the more technical aspect of the research.

Overview of outcomes, opportunities and challenges

Establishing and maintaining a forum of mixed members required careful preparation and on-going support meetings. The results of the study showed that community engagement can have a positive effect on the development, dissemination, and implementation of health research. Engaging with non-academic partners enables mutual learning and this also enhances the quality of NHS research.

This project team reported that community engagement could have a positive impact on the development, dissemination, and implementation of health research. Evaluations from members of the forum suggested that they enjoyed being part of the action research group and found the experience valuable in their professional roles. The authors stated that the engagement with non-academic partners enabled mutual learning. The researchers learned about the relevance of topics and importance of outcomes which were meaningful to the range of users and their mutual learning, therefore, enhanced the quality of National Health Service (NHS) research.

Creating the social conditions for the forum was, however, challenging, because of the heterogeneous nature of the group. The research team found the experiential knowledge of participants invaluable in discussing the focus of the research messages and the practical implications. Ideas from the group on dissemination outlets were rich, practical, and very useful. Individuals had come with varying expectations and perspectives. Maintaining the forum was also a challenge, in particular, securing the continuous attendance of statutory sector members. In addition there were problems with the attendance of the members of the forum in that only 7 out of the 12 members attended all three meetings. The authors reported that the Local Primary Care Trust members did not attend and that the initial resistance from social services to engage with the forum hindered recruitment to it for some time.

Example 4.2   How to use participatory action research in primary care (Marincowitz, 2003)

The aim of this study was to demonstrate the usefulness of Participatory Action Research (PAR) in Primary Care. It was conducted in Southern Africa.

Rationale for carrying out an action research project

The author wished to develop a deeper understanding of mutual participation in doctor–patient encounters and, secondly, to apply this learning in a rural cross-cultural setting. The basic structure of PAR has been described as an 'ever increasing spiral process of planning, acting, observing, reflecting, developing theory and re-planning'. The author stated that participation, collaboration, and the mutuality of all participants on all levels of the research were the ideal in all stages – identifying the problem, defining the problem, planning the research, collecting the data, interpreting the data, planning the intervention, evaluating the intervention, and re-evaluating the problem in light of the new information generated from the action and implementing and finally disseminating the information. Equality in sharing control and power was described as a basic value of PAR.

Background

In this study, PAR was undertaken with four patient groups. Four patients with a terminal illness formed groups with their family members, friends, and neighbours. Seven meetings with each group were audio-taped over the research period of six months. Each group consisted of the primary patient, the author (and research facilitator) who was their regular doctor, plus family members, friends, and neighbours. In three of the groups, a home-based care volunteer also formed part of the group. The number of people in each of the groups ranged from four to eight.

Action phase

The group met on a monthly basis. The author facilitated the meetings and acted as the research facilitator for all four groups. The meetings were conducted in Tsonga, the first language of the participants (the author was also fluent in Tsonga). The author kept a reflective diary and another member of the group made a written record of each meeting. Three free attitude interviews were also conducted with the author during this period. All the meetings were audio-taped. These took place in the patient participants' homes. During the first meeting, the purpose of the research was explained by the researcher with the statement: 'I want you to help me to understand better how we can work together as partners to improve the life of the patient, in view of the fact that his/her condition is incurable and chronic ... I may have scientific knowledge, but I do not know how it should be applied to a specific person's life because each person is different and this knowledge will work differently for each person'. Each group was encouraged to give ideas on patient management. Action plans were formulated and tried out. Decisions were made by the common consensus of the whole group. Data analysis was carried out by the researcher, due to language issues, but any summaries and themes were shared with the group for elaboration and clarification.

Outcomes

The PAR process had a positive effect on the doctor-patient encounter. The patients who participated benefitted the most. The reflective diary, which the author kept throughout the research period, recorded what happened during their research meetings, any communications with others about the patient and his/her illness, as well as thoughts about the concepts and processes that were relevant to the research topic. Based on the themes which emerged, a model was constructed which demonstrated the interrelatedness of different themes.

Researchers' comments on action research as a methodology

The author maintained that PAR was very applicable in Primary Care. The principles of PAR – such as mutual collaboration, reciprocal respect, co-learning, and acting on results from the enquiry – were all essential in the doctor-patient relationship. Skills of self-awareness, the ability to reflect, and keeping a reflective diary also had the potential to nurture the development of Primary Care workers.

Summary

We started this chapter by highlighting the benefits gained by healthcare professionals through undertaking action research projects. We suggested that it would be worthwhile for researchers to be aware of issues of quality while planning a project and a set of quality criteria was presented. The various contexts for undertaking action research were discussed. In the second half of the chapter we offered extensive guidance to the reader on the various stages for carrying out action research projects. Advice was provided on the selection of a research topic, its refinement, and revision, resulting from discussions with colleagues and planning action and evaluations. A planning grid was presented to support the researcher. We discussed how an action researcher may need to take into account 'what might go wrong' in the course of an inquiry. In the concluding section we offered practical examples of action research and invited the reader to plan a project.

Further reading

Hart, E. and Bond, M. (1995) *Action Research for Health and Social Care*. London: Open University Press.

McNiff, J. and Whitehead, J. (2005) *All You Need To Know About Action Research*. London: SAGE.

Meyer, J. (2006) 'Action research', in K. Gerrish and A. Lacey (eds), *The Research Process in Nursing*. Oxford: Blackwell.

Reason, P. and Bradbury, H. (2008) *The SAGE Handbook of Action Research: Participative Inquiry and Practice* (2nd edition). London: SAGE.

Stringer, E.T. and Genat, W.J. (2004) *Action Research in Health*. Upper Saddle River, NJ: Pearson Prentice-Hall.

Waterman, H., Tillen, D., Dickson, R. and de Koning, K. (2001) 'Action research: a systematic review and assessment for guidance', *Health Technology Assessment, 5* (23).

Welsh Assembly Government (2007) *Action Research Resource Pack*. Available from www.wales.gov.uk/cmoresearch

Whitelaw, S., Beattie, A., Balogh, R. and Watson, J. (2003) *A Review of the Nature of Action Research*. Cardiff: Welsh Assembly Government.

Winter, R. and Munn-Giddings, C. (2001) *A Handbook for Action Research in Health and Social Care*. London: Routledge.

5

Gathering Data

This chapter focuses on:

- Aspects of methodology
- Ethical considerations
- Methods of data collection and the relative advantages and possible disadvantages of these
- Quality issues.

Introduction

All researchers need to make decisions about which methodology to use in their research. In a research inquiry, researchers would have made the decision to use an action research approach. Some consideration may have been given to which data would need to be collected. The reader may have been asking two questions: what methods should a researcher be using and how should they go about organizing the data collection? If a researcher is working for an academic qualification they may have also been attending lectures on research methodology in an academic institution. In this chapter we shall focus on aspects of data gathering in some detail; our aim is to provide an overview of the methodological issues and to discuss the most commonly used methods in action research. Our focus is on the practical aspects of the processes of data collection. The relative advantages and possible disadvantages of various methods of data collection are discussed. As it is not possible to cover all the aspects of data collection within this introductory text, we have provided further reading at the end of the chapter for any further study.

In the context of collecting and using data, researchers need to be aware of an important difference between traditional research and action research. When conducting action research the data are gathered, analysed, and reflected on throughout the project – and the emerging findings are shared with all the participants and used to refine any action. This is not always the case with other forms of research.

Making a start

A useful exercise for an action researcher to be engaged in, at this stage, is to read three or four published papers which report on action research projects. The reader may wish to use full versions of some of the papers we have included in this book, or access new ones which may share similar objectives to any inquiry the reader is interested in. Taking note of what data researchers have collected and the methods they used to gather them is worthwhile. A critical eye in appraising what has been presented is also of value. Researchers should ask some general questions at this stage such as: what are the objectives of the project and do the sources of data generate evidence to support the achievement of the declared objectives? Also, are the data collection methods practical and feasible? It may help researchers to use the grid in Table 5.1 to get started on the data collection process, working in pairs or groups.

TABLE 5.1   *A review of data collection in action research projects*

Short title of the paper, author, and date of publication	Objectives of the research or research questions	Data sets
Paper 1	To improve ...	e.g. semi-structured interviews, focus groups, questionnaires, personal research journals
Paper 2		
Paper 3		
Paper 4		

Researchers should complete the details in the grid and then consider the following questions, for each of the papers, in some detail, by sharing their views on the process of data collection. In the true spirit of action research, working in groups can both enhance the quality of discussions and the decisions made with reference to the data-gathering for a project:

- What is the topic of research or the research question?
- What is the overall aim in carrying out this study?
- What are the specific objectives of the study?
- What constitutes the 'action' stage?
- What kind of evidence is needed for monitoring and evaluating the actions?
- Can the gathered data provide what is required?

- Who is to collect the data?
- From whom will the data be collected?
- Have ethical issues been addressed?
- How are the data to be managed and processed?
- Do the data-gathering methods sound feasible within the time-scale of the project?

Researchers should give some of their discussion time to considering the research questions or objectives and how these relate to the data collection methods of the project. This is because the main purpose of collecting data is to generate evidence to find out what action to take or to understand the impact of what it is the researchers are aiming to achieve. Asking the right questions is of paramount importance in all research and action research is no exception.

Methodological issues

Before considering any methods of data collection it would be useful for researchers to revisit the discussion we had previously on the philosophical underpinning necessary in the context of action research, in terms of ontological and epistemological considerations. Ontology is the nature of being or what entities can be said to exist. Epistemology (the theory of knowledge) is concerned with our beliefs about what it is possible to know – whether we believe that the 'absolute truth' can ever be known. It is important for researchers to state their philosophical position as this is known within the research design, as data collection and analysis will be influenced by personal attitudes and beliefs. If they are carrying out research as part of obtaining a qualification, researchers will certainly need to demonstrate some knowledge of different research paradigms and associated worldviews. An elaborate discussion of different paradigms of research is beyond the scope of this book, so if a study is leading to a dissertation a researcher would need to do some supplementary reading which would be provided in research methods lectures and from the further reading listed at the end of this chapter.

To begin with, the overarching paradigm or worldview of action research would need to be stated. The reader will recall the discussions on the theoretical underpinnings of action research. So by way of an extension of the discussion in Chapter 1, we have listed the key features of each of the three paradigms below. These can be used as a justification for the approach researchers wish to take. So, for example, a key feature of critical theory is to promote social justice and therefore it can be used to support an action research project which aims to empower people to take control and change their situation for the better. Or researchers might want to use an interpretive paradigm because they want to utilize a process of deep attentiveness and empathetic understanding via a close examination of the perceptions of staff

TABLE 5.2   *Key features of the three major paradigms found in action research (adapted from Guba and Lincoln, 2005)*

Paradigm Feature	Interpretive	Critical	Participatory
Goal	Better understanding of people's situations	Seeks the abolition of social injustice. Aims to improve the social situations of those who are experiencing the problem being studied.	Transforms the world in the service of human flourishing.
Ontology	Mulitiple realities, constructed and holistic. Humans actively construct their own meanings of situations.	Realities are shaped over time by social, politicial, cultural economic, ethnic, and gender values.	Subjective–objective reality.
Epistemology	Meaning arises out of social situations and is handled through interpretive processes. Data are socially situated, context-related, context-dependent, and context-rich. Knower and known are interactive and inseparable.	Findings are assessed in the light of a particular value–system, objectivity and subjectivity are both valued.	Extended epistemology of experiential, imaginal, propositional and practical knowing (see Figure 5.1.).
Values	Included and seen to be formative.	Included and seen to be very important in determining action.	Included and seen to be formative.
Knowledge accumulation	Generalizability is interpreted as generalizability to identifiable, specific settings and subjects rather than universally.	Knowledge is historically situated according to the context of the time.	In communities of inquiry embedded in communities of practice.

and patients 'from the inside'. Or perhaps a participatory paradigm might be more appealing if researchers are particularly interested in promoting patient participation in care. Table 5.2 should illuminate these ideas for the reader.

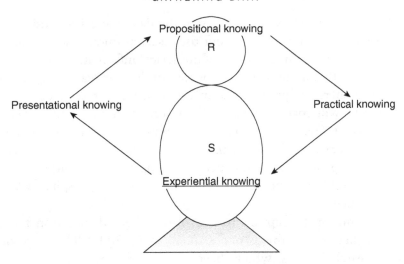

FIGURE 5.1   *The circuit of fourfold knowing (Heron, 1996: 53).*

It is quite possible to carry out quantatitive or qualitative research methods in any of these paradigms, as they are merely research methods to achieve goals despite the fact that traditionally quantitative research comes from a positivist and qualitative research from an interpretive paradigm. As we suggested earlier it is up to the action researcher and the team to decide which paradigm they will follow.

Quantitative and qualitative data

Action researchers should also consider the usefulness of quantitative and qualitative research within the context of their work. Action research uses a variety of paradigms and researchers need to have justified for themselves what it is they are interested in. Quantitative data are measured and represented by numbers whereas qualitative research attempts to gain insights into the experiences and behaviours of subjects in specific contexts. Data generated within a qualitative approach will be based on interactions and the interpretations of these made by researchers. When researchers handle large amounts of data – for example, a large number of questionnaires, surveys, tests results – it is often necessary to analyse them using statistical methods and then to present these in the form of tables and charts. If researchers are collecting views using questionnaires from a relatively small group of colleagues or patients about their perceptions or attitudes, they may still wish to represent the data numerically using tables and charts in the action research, but the research findings are unlikely to be based simply on a small amount of numerical information. What we can say, however, is that in most of the reported studies the reader will find that action researchers are predominantly using qualitative research methods and the data will mainly consist of transcripts of in-depth interviews, observations of practice, descriptions of outcomes of meetings, entries in personal journals, field notes, and documentary analysis, which enable researchers to gain insights into people's behaviours and interactions in their natural settings, whether this is in health clinics, hospital wards, or general practice.

It is a common perception that all data collected in action research will be qualitative but this is not so (Gall et al., 2007). There are many action research studies which have used questionnaire surveys and numerical data. For example, Hampshire et al. (1999) report on the use of a mixture of qualitative and quantitative data collection methods, which included the administration of questionnaires with 534 parents in their research design. They used the SPSS computer software for data analysis and tested the results for statistical significance. In their study they also used a pre- and post-project design for assessing the effectiveness of their action research project and also set up a comparison group. A pre-post design to assess the effectiveness of an intervention may be criticized as it is inherently weak in determining causality. All action researchers using this design would need to discuss this.

Qualitative data are not inferior in status and, in action research, these have the added appeal in that they can illuminate human feelings and provide rich insights into actions and their consequences. What is important is to select the type of data which will serve the purpose of a study. As most of the action research studies we have reviewed used qualitative research methods, we will now consider the attributes of qualitative research in greater detail.

Ethical considerations

When researchers are carrying out research it is important they follow ethical guidelines. If this research is based in an academic institution there would be a set of institutional guidelines for ethical approval for researchers to follow. Ethical approval from the National Health Service is required for all research involving patients. Most health professional bodies, such as

The Royal College of Nursing, will provide their own ethical guidelines and the Research Governance Framework (Department of Health, 2005) sets out the standards for the NHS. For action research to be carried out in local contexts, researchers will most probably be applying to local ethics approval committees. Reading the guidelines on ethics published by these authoritative sources is a useful starting point.

Although the general principles apply to all research, for action research projects the ethical implications and procedures will be slightly different. On the one hand, as action research projects are not designed to carry out experiments with different treatments or drug trials they do not have control groups which are treated differently thus making ethical procedures less complex. However, on the other hand, action researchers face a different but complex dimension to ethical issues. As action research is quite often carried out as small-scale projects and located within the working situations of researchers, special care needs to be taken both for data collection and the dissemination of findings as it can be easy to recognize people and events within local situations. Another problem that action researchers may face is that the changing direction of the research as action is continually informed by data collection and analysis which means new ethical issues may arise and these will need to be dealt with.

Although it is not possible to include all aspects of the ethical requirements for action research projects in this book, the reader may find the following guidance helpful. We start with what Winter and Munn-Giddings (2001: 220) highlight as the important principles which should guide action researchers in their professional contexts. These are:

- the duty of care (which overrides mere personal interest);
- respect for the individual, irrespective of race, gender, age, disability, etc.;
- respect for cultural diversity;
- respect for individual dignity;
- protection from harm.

The National Research Ethics Service has also published guidelines on user involvement in research which provide useful advice on ethics concerning participatory research (PR) and since action research is PR this is highly pertinent (see http://www.nres.npsa.nhs.uk/patients-and-the-public/public-involvement-in-research). We would strongly urge the reader to examine these prior to submitting an ethics application. Below is a list of ethical considerations for adoption when involving users (patients and staff) in research.

- Provide jargon free-information on the research.
- Provide additional information on which training will be involved, what the role of users will entail, and how they will be supported.
- Give 24 hours for individuals to make up their minds to participate.
- Do not coerce or over incentivize people to take part.
- Inform them that they have the right to withdraw at any time from the research without explanation.
- Take written or tape recorded consent prior and during the study.
- Identify, explain, and minimize the burdens and risks of participating in an action research project. These will result from the time and emotional investment needed.
- Have a plan of action if participants should become distressed during meetings.
- Promote a culture of confidentiality amongst the participants by agreeing on ground rules for behaviour within the group.
- Undertake risk assessments of their safety.

The last point which refers to the safety of researchers can become an issue if, for example, a user leaves their usual environment to travel externally to an interview or meeting. To overcome this potential problem, researchers may need training in risk assessment, including on how to use safety technology, how to de-escalate potentially dangerous situations, and how to respond. Below are some tips on how researchers may increase their safety on external visits.

- Beforehand, an assessment of the risk should be made and if this is high it should be discussed with the supervisor/manager.
- A researcher must speak to the person beforehand, give them their work details so they will expect them, and confirm these by letter or e-mail later.
- If a researcher is using electronic safety devices, they must make sure they know how to operate these and that the batteries are charged before they leave.
- A researcher must ring to remind the interviewee on the day of interview and wear appropriate clothing and jewellery.
- A researcher must be aware of the nearest exit in the interview room and must not let the interviewee sit between them and it.
- A researcher should follow local policy on who to leave details of the date and time of interview with, the contact numbers, the make of car if appropriate, the person and their address, the time at which they expect to finish the interview, and the nearest police station.
- If a researcher is upset as a result of the interview, they should discuss this with an appropriate person, for example, a supervisor.
- The designated safety person must follow local policy on their responsibilities if a researcher does not check in.
- The researcher must ring in at the specified time.
- If an adverse incident occurs, it should be reported immediately and the local policy must be followed.

(Adapted from the policy of the School of Nursing, Midwifery and Social Work, University of Manchester)

Addressing ethical issues

Participant Information Sheet

A Participant Information Sheet (PIS) should be made available to all prospective collaborators and participants. The sheet should state the purpose of the project, why the participants have been invited to join, and their roles, as well as any benefits and possible disadvantages to joining the project. In an action research project which is designed to improve aspects of practice, it is unlikely researchers will face resistance from invited participants. The PIS should include details of how the data and any findings will be used during and at the end of the project. In an action research project it is also important that researchers explain how the data and interpretations will be shared with participants. Assurances should be given that all the information gathered during the project will be kept confidential by keeping the names and identities of co-researchers unrecognizable. The name of a contact person should also be given, who will be available to discuss any issues about the project at any time during it. Researchers must give ample time for all the participants to study the information and must be prepared to answer any further questions and alleviate any anxieties and misunderstandings. The PIS should be written in a style which is easily understood and avoids jargon. If participants have reading or language difficulties, arrangements should be made for making the PIS accessible.

Informed consent

Informed consent must be obtained from all participants. A consent form can be distributed at the same time as the PIS. This should make it clear that participation is voluntary and that the participants can withdraw from the study at any time. Researchers should explain what the study involves and what their respective roles are. Participation should be voluntary and no one should feel they must participate in the project. This can be an issue when an academic facilitator or a manager invites participants to take part (as they may feel pressurized to join the project either because they are his or her students or because they see the leader as their superior and are concerned about the consequences of declining the offer to join). To prevent feelings of coercion sometimes it is helpful to engage an independent person to take the consents. Parents/guardians will also have to be consulted if children or people who may have a disability are being invited to participate. Written permission should be sought for publishing people's views at all stages of the research. As the course of an action research project is unpredictable, it is wise to reaffirm consent at regular intervals (say, every meeting) to make sure participants are still comfortable with being part of that project.

Other issues

As previously stated, Winter and Munn-Giddings (2001) list some ethical issues, specific to action research projects, which will also need to be addressed. One is protection from harm. Participants in the project may need to talk about emotionally difficult issues or take part in discussions with people representing roles which they feel suspicious about and where conflicting opinions may be voiced. These may result in painful experiences and the participants have a right to expect the process to have been planned in such a way that such pain is minimized and support is available if it occurs. The other issue they highlight is, as in all research, the ethical duty to be honest in the reporting of data and analysing and drawing conclusions from these. The need to listen to the voices of all participants at all stages is also stressed.

Details of how ethical issues are to be addressed within an action research project will need to be included in any proposals and most certainly before a project starts. Authors of academic dissertations and doctoral theses will be expected to address ethical issues in their work. Published papers using action research as an approach will usually include a section on ethical considerations, which tends to be shorter in length due to the word limits prescribed for journal submissions. The following extract, outlining how ethical issues were addressed in a project based in a developing country, was taken from an article published in the *International Journal of Mental Health Nursing*. Full details can be found in the references at the end of this book.

Example 5.1   Introducing peer-group clinical supervision: an action research project (Lakeman and Glasgow, 2009)

Approval for undertaking this project was obtained from the Dublin City University Human Research Ethics Committee (Dublin, Ireland) and the hospital nursing administration. Concern was raised by the ethics committee, regarding how sustainable the project might be in a developing country (i.e. whether the supervision would continue after the research phase was completed). This was addressed by assurances that the project would be ongoing for as long as people were willing to participate (one researcher was employed in the hospital and could make this commitment) and noting that participants were in a sense co-researchers rather than subjects. Potential participants were provided with information sheets relating to the project and returned a consent form at a later date, if they chose to participate (minimizing the potential for any pressure or coercion to participate).

Methods of data collection

In the following section, we will look at the methods for data collection which are commonly used within action research. Before exploring these, we will provide the reader with two important points which all researchers should usefully bear in mind when planning data collection. First, there are many ways to gather data; researchers must choose the most suitable method for the research objectives or questions and, secondly, the quality of the data collected is more important than the number of ways the information is collected. It should be useful at this stage for researchers to further reflect on the following aspects:

- the nature of the evidence researchers need to collect to achieve the aims of the study;
- the time-scale for data-gathering;
- the total time available to carry out the project;
- the usefulness of the data which researchers intend to collect;
- a consideration of how researchers may analyse and interpret the data.

As we present a variety of data-gathering methods commonly used within action research, we will also try to provide general guidance on the procedures, their relative merits and any possible disadvantages that researchers need to bear in mind. Further reading on data collection methods is provided at the end of this chapter.

A review of the different data gathering methods used by action researchers showed that these range from using a single open-ended question to gather information (as is the case in a study by Van Deventer and Hugo, 2005, who conducted a listening survery with a single open question 'What is happening in this village?') to data gathering using a mixture of methods which can be seen in the following summary extract, from a journal article which reported on an action research study that was designed to improve patients' experience at mealtimes in a hospital ward. Full details are provided in the reference section at the end of this book.

Hospital mealtimes: action research for change (Dickinson et al., 2005)

The methods included the use of focus groups, interviews, observation, and benchmarking using the 'Essence of Care' benchmarking tool from the Department of Health (2001).

(Continued)

(Continued)

Focus groups

Focus groups, i.e. group discussions that focus on a specific set of issues can capture different perspectives and views about a specific experience or event (Kreuger, 1994) and group members are able to respond to and discuss each others' comments, as well as 'tease out previously taken for granted assumptions' (Bloor et al., 2001).

Focus group discussions were held at the beginning of the project, before the action research intervention began, in order to identify the difficulties with mealtimes and nutrition-related work on the unit, and these were to be repeated at the end of the implementation phase. The focus group included members of staff working on the unit, with representations from healthcare assistants, qualified nursing staff, and occupational therapy and physiotherapy staff. Photographs representing mealtimes on the unit were shown to participants as a stimulus to promote discussions at the beginning of the focus groups while the questions used in the groups focused on various aspects of the mealtime experience. These groups were held in a quiet room and were conducted by two researchers, with one researcher taking notes while the other researcher facilitated the discussion. Three focus groups involving 19 staff were undertaken and were tape-recorded and transcribed.

Interviews with patients

Qualitative interviews, with a flexible structure based on a series of open-ended questions constructed to cover the subject being researched, were undertaken. The interviews were used to help see the mealtime from a patient perspective and to explore patients' experiences and views of the unit mealtimes. Six patients in total were interviewed.

Observations

Six mealtimes were observed. All three mealtimes were included in the observations, and each was observed by two individuals, enabling all the geographical areas of the unit to be included. Observations, which included the location of eating, the involvement and activity of nursing staff, and the timing and duration of events were recorded onto an observational schedule designed for the project.

The methods of data collection used in the above example will be examined in the next section of this chapter. These cover:

- interviews;
- focus groups;
- the use of questionnaires;

- the use of field diaries and personal reflective journals;
- gathering documentary evidence;
- recording Critical (Significant) Incidents.

Conducting interviews

Interviews are the most common method used by action researchers. The reason for this, perhaps, is best reflected in the opening paragraph of Kvale and Brinkmann's recent book:

> If you want to know how people understand their world and their lives, why not talk with them? ... Through conversations we get to know other people, learn about their experiences, feelings, attitudes and the world they live in. In an interview conversation, the researcher asks about, and listens to, what people themselves tell about their lived world. (2009: xvii)

The purpose of conducting interviews is in order to gather in-depth information about aspects of the research topic. Interviewing may be used as the single method of data collection or as a method to gather additional data when questionnaires and surveys are used.

Interviews may be conducted with individuals or in groups and there are different kinds. In a *structured interview,* the interviewer starts with a set of questions which are pre-determined and only these questions are asked. Responses to the questions from these interviews are easier to record as numerical data. In a *semi-structured interview,* the researcher prepares a set of questions, but also prepares a set of sub-questions which can be used to probe ideas further and gather more information. Researchers also have the option of using *open-ended interviews*. Semi-structured or open-question interviews are often used in action research as these can provide richer and more in-depth responses from participants. Semi-structured interviews allow researchers to follow different directions whilst retaining some control of the questions asked. Unstructured interviews can provide opportunities for gathering in-depth information and an open exploration of interviewees' viewpoints. There are still other kinds of interviews, such as group interviews, focus groups, and telephone interviews. Focus group interviews are discussed later in the chapter.

Some guidelines for researchers on individual interviews

- Check the location of the interviews before you set off.
- Carry out practice interviews and refine the questions as necessary (pilot interview questions when carrying out a structured interview).
- Select comfortable surroundings for the interview.
- Check the batteries and operation of the tape recorder.

- Explain the background to the study and the purpose of the interview at the start and assure anonymity. Establish a rapport. Remember to keep positive.
- Start with 'warm-up' questions to put interviewees at ease; ask any factual questions at the start.
- Prepare the questions and their sequence in advance; in some studies, participants are given the list of questions to enable them to think about their responses in advance.
- Give thinking time, accept silences, and don't rush the interview. Allow interviewees the opportunity to ask for a clarification of any questions asked. At the same time, keep to a reasonable pace.
- Make sure that the interviews are not too long (about 40 minutes to an hour should be about right).
- Semi-structured interviews allow researchers to probe during an interview, but have some idea about what this may cover and plan the questions in advance.
- Open-ended questions can often provide richer information. Asking participants to 'talk more about' something and using phrases such as 'that is interesting' can encourage them to open up and speak for longer. Try to repeat back their last words e.g. 'You felt sad … ?' as a prompt.
- Try not to convey any opinions during the interview.
- Avoid leading questions such as: 'Were you thinking about … when I asked you about … ? and 'Surely you think the right way is to … '
- Check for understanding by paraphrasing what interviewees have said.
- Ask interviewees if they have any questions at the end.

Advantages to carrying out interviews

- Interviews can often provide a relaxed context for the exploration of ideas.
- Information from interviews can supplement what has been gathered through questionnaires, surveys and observation.
- One-to-one interviews are useful for the exploration of sensitive issues.
- People who may not be confident enough to speak in larger groups are more likely to talk openly during an interview.
- The interviewer can steer the discussion through a fruitful route.
- Interviews can provide unexpected, but useful insights and perspectives.
- Interview transcripts can be used as powerful evidence when presenting data and during dissemination.
- Most interviewees will describe one-to-one interviews as a positive experience.

Possible disadvantages to carrying out interviews

- Conducting interviews can be more time-consuming than using questionnaires.
- Typing transcripts is labour intensive.
- Interviewing may not always be a suitable method to elicit views from those who are not confident speakers and those with language problems.
- The use of tape recorders may intimidate some people, so if they refuse to be recorded take notes instead that can be typed up afterwards.

- An interviewer's presence may make the interviewees nervous.
- An interviewee may only tell an interviewer what they think they want to hear.
- Tape-recording makes it possible for an interviewer to give their full attention to the context of the interview. Most interviews are tape recorded, but transcribing all of them would be time consuming if the numbers become large. An interviewer needs to make the choice whether they would listen to the tapes or read fully transcribed versions of the interviews when it is time to analyse these.

Focus groups

Focus groups were originally used for market research, but are increasingly being adopted for research in healthcare and social work. Focus group meetings can be very useful for exploring people's feelings, attitudes, beliefs, and views. They can provide insights into multiple perceptions, interactions, conflicting views, differences, and power issues. Focus groups will usually consist of six to ten members and the meeting is normally led by a facilitator or moderator. The facilitator allows participants to talk freely, expressing their views openly. The purpose is not to bring about agreements between participants on ideas, but to allow diverse viewpoints to be discussed. Focus group discussions are particularly suitable when controversial topics are discussed. They can be used as the only data-gathering method or can also be used to supplement data from other sources, such as questionnaires and surveys. Well facilitated group interactions can lead to discussions of aspects which may not otherwise be exposed. In addition the group situation can stimulate people into making explicit their views, perceptions, motives, and reasons. This makes group interviews an attractive data-gathering option when research is trying to probe those aspects in people's behaviour (Punch, 2009). Punch describes focus group interviews as data-rich, flexible, stimulating, recall-aiding, cumulative, and elaborative.

Describing the use of focus groups for data collection in their action research study Lakeman and Glasgow (2009) write:

> Focus groups were the main vehicles for data collection and collaborative decision making. Focus groups have particular usefulness in eliciting opinions and provoking participants to consider different opinions in the light of disclosures from others (Fontana & Fret, 2005). The focus groups proceeded in a semi-structured fashion involving the presentation of data from previous groups and a series of open-ended questions related to the current phase of the action research cycle (assessment, reflecting and planning). The focus group meetings were audio-taped and transcribed and used for content analysis.

Some guidelines for researchers on focus groups

- Keep the numbers small and manageable.
- Send reminders to encourage attendance.
- As the facilitator's role is crucial, make sure they have the requisite skills to lead the discussions.
- Remember to establish trust within the group.
- As is the case in all interviews, provide a comfortable environment and stay relaxed.
- Facilitators should avoid the temptation of disagreeing with the views of other members, which may be different to theirs.
- Having two people present in meetings may help, with one facilitator in a leading and moderating role and the other as a silent observer taking notes.
- Suggest some groundrules for speaking. For example, not talking over one another and addressing issues through the facilitator.
- Summarizing what has been said before at different points can help to elicit different viewpoints.
- Watch out for those individuals who will tend to dominate the discussion and try to make sure everyone has a turn.
- It is important to be aware of the nature of the group. Some participants may be reluctant to share their thoughts in the company of their managers and certain stakeholders.
- It may be necessary to pay travel and other costs to the participants.
- Focus group discussions can provide opportunities for members to revise their views and perspectives during and after meetings.
- The discussions can enhance participants' understanding of issues relating to the topic of inquiry.

Advantages to using focus groups

- Focus groups can provide a quicker method for gathering viewpoints and comments than conducting individual interviews.
- They can give a flexible approach to steering conversations and directions.
- They can act as a forum where conflicting views can be expressed.
- Used with other methods, they can supplement the information already collected.
- They can be more time-saving than individual interviews.
- Some people prefer discussions in groups as they will feel less threatened than when being interviewed individually and focus groups can supply this.

Possible disadvantages to using focus groups

- Poor attendance.
- The success of focus group discussions will depend on the skills and experience of the moderator/facilitator. Selecting the right person can be a challenge.
- Some members may feel threatened by the composition of the group in terms of power relationships and may choose not to contribute.

- Members may be shy or might lack the confidence to speak in large groups.
- People with language problems may not be able to communicate their thoughts easily.
- Transcribing group discussions can sometimes be challenging.
- There may be a tendency for members to agree with the views of others, rather than disagree and create tensions.
- Analysis of the data generated from focus groups may be more complex.
- Organizing meetings can sometimes be time consuming.
- The facilitator's bias may influence discussions.

Questionnaires

Some action research studies will use questionnaires, but these are rarely adopted as the only method for collecting data. They can sometimes be used at the start of a project to gather initial thoughts and perceptions and these are then supplemented by other data-gathering methods. As most action research projects are small scale in nature, using questionnaires may not be the most effective way to gather vital information. And as the nature of action research is participative and collaborative, asking participants to complete questionnaires may not be perceived as being compatible with the true spirit of the action research approach.

Questionnaires can be useful when researchers wish to collect a range of information – say when consulting a larger group of patients or health workers in clinical settings – with relative ease; these can then be followed up as necessary. For example, if an action research project involves the introduction of a new way of working, it may help researchers to use a questionnaire to provide them with simple means to collect information about what is happening before planning an intervention. The completed questionnaires can help in two ways. They can provide data on perceptions, attitudes, and behaviours before any intervention begins. And secondly, the analysis of the questionnaire responses may help to shape the nature of the questions researchers may want to ask during individual interviews – to decide on the content of focus group discussions or to structure any observations they may wish to conduct. Within a questionnaire, researchers can use both short questions and open-ended questions which will need fuller responses.

Some guidelines for researchers on using questionnaires
Here is a set of guidelines that may prove useful:

- Open-ended questions are likely to provide richer and more meaningful data, although they may also deter people from responding and can be more difficult to analyse.
- Keep the questionnaire simple. By designing appropriate questions, this can often produce a decent amount of data, just by using a small number of questions.

- Consider how the responses to the questions can be analysed when designing the questions.
- Start with questions about any factual information required.
- Use clear, simple language which all the respondents will understand and avoid any jargon.
- Avoid leading questions. For example, a question such as 'Which part of the day do you find the most difficult to manage?' assumes that the respondent does indeed find a part of the day difficult to manage – which may not be the case.
- Emphasize the anonymity of the responses.
- Consult a statistician who can advise on how to analyse the data.
- Do a pilot run before giving out questionnaires and make any adjustments as necessary. Acknowledge, in the final report, this pilot effort and any changes that were made to the final version of the questionnaire.
- Take account of those who may have language difficulties when administering a questionnaire – it may be necessary to use translated versions.

Advantages to using questionnaires

- They enable researchers to collect background information fairly easily.
- They can help researchers to gather a reasonable amount of data in a short time.
- They can provide information which can be followed up.
- They can provide numerical information which is easy to represent in frequencies as displays.

Possible disadvantages to using questionnaires

- Researchers may be subjective and introduce bias in the type of questions they ask.
- Responses may be influenced by what the respondents believe researchers want to hear.
- Designing a questionnaire needs great skill, especially when using open-ended questions which are designed to be probing. Researchers must take note of the previous section about the challenges involving the analysis of open-ended questions.
- If researchers are using questionnaires in order to collect data from a larger group of people who are not within their institution, returns and response rates may be too low to ensure a valid research outcome.

Field diaries and personal reflective journals

The use of a research diary or a personal reflective journal, as it is sometimes referred to, is a very helpful method for recording information during an action research project. This is used for keeping a record of what happens and where any ideas evolve from, as well as the research process itself. It is a document where a researcher can write down their experiences and thoughts as they occur. It is also a place where they would keep an account of their reflections and write a personal commentary on their feelings, as well as any emerging interpretations. A research diary could be extremely valuable when it comes to writing up a project, as it contains the authentic voice of the researcher as described throughout the research process. The reflective process involved in writing a diary can also contribute to the professional development of a researcher. Diary entries need not be very long, but should include accounts of events and the developing understanding of issues. It becomes a log of a personal journey during the project. At the start of the project, a researcher will be keeping an account of what happens as events unfold, but as the journal progresses they would start to interpret the entries and notice the emerging themes.

Winter and Munn–Giddings (2001) explain the purpose and usefulness of keeping research dairies under five headings, which are summarized below:

- *For creating a database of events, experiences, and thoughts*
  The researcher needs to make detailed notes as things occur and ideas as they 'strike' without waiting for them to fall into a clear and significant pattern. Unless these are recorded at the time they may be forgotten, and it is precisely those experiences and thoughts that don't immediately fit into what is expected that are the growth points for new thinking. Unless these are written down in detail at the time, researchers will only remember them selectively in a way which fits into familiar lines of thought and neglects the aspects that were unexpected.
- *For creating a collaborative basis for reflection*
  It is better for as many participants as possible to keep personal diaries. If only one person keeps a diary undue prominence will gradually be given to that person's ideas, which goes against the collaborative spirit of action research. If more researchers keep diaries, the differing perspectives will be created and documented and these can be compared as part of the reflective process.
- *As a way of keeping a train of thought alive*
  It is advisable for researchers to set aside a regular time for making entries in their research diary, but unexpected ideas may 'pop up' which also should be recorded. The diary is a convenient way of keeping one part of the mind creatively occupied with the research, without a researcher necessarily being aware of it. Keeping spare pieces of paper at all times so that entries can be made as they become alive is one way of achieving this.
- *As the source for a document that can be shared with others*
  If a researcher's thinking becomes 'stuck' in rather familiar lines, one way of starting a new line of thought is to show some extracts from a diary to other participants or the action research group leader. This is a useful way of gaining new perspectives and other possible ways to think about events.
- *As notes for any final report*
  The diary will provide a range of material when it comes to writing up the project without having to start from scratch.

Some guidelines for researchers on keeping a research diary or personal journal

- Keep the diary in a safe place so as to keep the contents confidential.
- Use a loose-leaf file.
- Record the date and time to show the development of any thinking and progress on the project.
- Use a free writing style.
- It is useful to have a structure in mind. Within that structure, include the flexibility to make notes about those aspects which may not fit into the predetermined structure, as these may become significant at a later stage.
- Reflective writing supports professional development. Try to be analytical and reflective in each entry.
- Using different colours to mark any emerging themes can be helpful.
- Sharing the diary with someone who is not involved in the research can help with personal reflection. However, do be careful about confidentiality!
- Including a section for personal commentary can support analysis and discussions at a later stage.

Advantages to keeping field diaries and journals

- Keeping a research diary helps to personalize researcher involvement in the project.
- They can help to keep a progress check on the project.
- Field diaries can often supplement information obtained from other sources.
- The process of personal reflective writing is an integral part of professional development.
- The contents of a diary should help researchers to construct the research story at the time of writing up.

Possible disadvantages to keeping field diaries and journals

- A researcher may be tempted to write too much, which can lead to difficulties at the time of analysis.
- It is sometimes difficult to keep up with the writing regularly due to the pressure of other work.
- When the research does not appear to be going according to plan, there may be a tendency for researchers to stop writing.
- Personalizing the entries and incidents may introduce a higher level of subjectivity into the accounts.

Systematic observation

Systematic observation is sometimes used in action research projects for data-gathering. Observation is a natural process – we observe people and incidents all the time and, based on those observations, we make judgements.

Basically, we are making use of this within the research process, where there will be a need for more systematic observation, so that the information we collect can be used for the purpose of the study. In practical terms, it involves researchers recording what they see. Observations can be made of situations, events, behaviours, and interactions between people. Carrying out observations needs considerable skill in recording what is going on. In healthcare settings, gathering information through observation requires a high level of sensitivity. The context of the observations needs to be explained and the sequence of activities accurately described.

When we consider observation as a method for data collection, two types are often commonly referred to: participant and non-participant observation. *Participant observation* involves the researcher living in the context and being a part of it, but they need to be aware of their biases in what they record and interpret (Cohen and Manion, 1994). The researcher needs to be conscious of this and acknowledge it. Therefore there is a possibility of introducing what one wishes to see in the data gathered. This could distort the interpretations made from observational data. *Non-participant observation* involves observing actions and interactions, perhaps sitting in a corner of the room, silent but attentive. Both types of observation require careful planning.

The nature and purpose of the observation process will influence the level of structuring researchers need to introduce. Through structured observations, they can gather both qualitative and quantitative data. Using carefully designed observation schedules, researchers can record behaviour patterns and the number of actions and interactions. In semi-structured observation procedures they may still use pre-defined schedules, but some flexibility should be built in to enable researchers to record any unexpected outcomes which may also be of some value. As data from observations are likely to be more subjective, having more than one person observing can achieve greater objectivity in the procedure.

Some guidelines for researchers on the use of observation

- Decide who is going to be a participant or non-participant observer before the structure of the observations is planned.
- Structured observation schedules can be useful. This may be an established structure or one that is designed for the purpose in hand.
- If using a pre-determined observation schedule, researchers need to allow the flexibility to record unexpected outcomes which could be of significance within the context of a project. Try a pilot observation and refine the process as necessary.
- Consider access and time-scales for the observations.

- Ethically as a clinician, as well as a researcher, it is important to discuss with those being studied how a researcher will react if someone needs their immediate assistance in the case of an emergency or if they witness malpractice.
- Give some thought to the process of data analysis, while preparing the observation schedules.
- Consider how the observations will be validated.
- Make a note of any difficulties encountered as these may be of significance when analysing the data and writing up your report.

Advantages to using observation

- First-hand information is collected, as the events happen, based on what is actually seen and heard.
- Open-ended observations with little or no structure allow for the capture of all aspects of the topic under study.
- It offers a way of studying contexts and behaviour, through close scrutiny.
- Observations can provide researchers with opportunities to take note of reactions (boredom, frustration, and disinterest for example) which may also be of value in the construction of the research narrative.
- If using a video recorder, the observation can be replayed as many times as necessary.

Possible disadvantages to using observation

- Observations can cause disruption in a setting, for example in a hospital ward or care home.
- If more than one person is involved in carrying out the observation, it may be difficult to reach a consensus on what has been observed.
- What is being written down may be affected by researchers' own beliefs and perceptions.
- It can be very time-consuming.
- Too much information may be collected which could pose a challenge for any analysis.
- Being observed may affect the behaviour of the persons observed.
- Organizational problems may stand in the way of carrying out observations effectively.
- Background noise and disruptions may lead to researchers missing important data.
- Researchers may need to contend with tricky ethical issues concerning the type and level of intervention in emergencies and in cases of malpractice.

Using video and DVD recordings for observations

The use of videos and DVDs to record events is becoming increasingly popular as a data-gathering technique. The availability of digital cameras and other technological resources has made recording a viable and effective way of gathering information. One of the advantages of video recording is that it allows the researcher to observe an activity afterwards by watching the video. By viewing recordings researchers will be able to analyse different aspects of the activity, as well as identify any unexpected aspects which may be significant.

Advantages to video/DVD recording

- Actions, behaviours, and attitudes can be captured with greater accuracy than by making observation notes.
- Provides a more permanent record of incidents which can be viewed and re-viewed.
- Makes sharing data with colleagues and fellow researchers easier to manage.
- Can be useful at the time of dissemination. Recording provides powerful images which are hard to match through other means of communication.
- Video and film clips can often generate a good deal of discussion between observers and audiences with whom researchers will be sharing their findings.

Possible disadvantages to recording events

- Expensive to purchase equipment.
- Video recording might miss important data off screen.
- Being recorded can be inhibiting and distracting for the participants.
- Those who are being recorded may behave differently in the presence of a camera.
- Technical hitches may lose useful first-hand data which cannot be replaced.
- The transcription of videos can prove painstaking.

Gathering documentary evidence

In some cases the data collection would include studying documentary evidence such as local health policies, the minutes of meetings, and other records to supplement other data sources. These can often provide a useful background and context for a project and can also be very illuminating.

Advantages to gathering documentary evidence

- Documentary evidence can provide insights into the situation where the research is taking place.
- In most cases it can provide information without too much effort.
- A record of objectives and policies which are not easily communicated can be accessed through documents.
- It can support other forms of evidence that have been collected.

Possible disadvantages to collecting documentary evidence

- Trust in the researcher will be necessary before access to documents is given.
- It may constitute large amounts of data, so selection and analysis could be difficult.
- Personal choices may affect the type of documents collected.
- Not all the information that is needed might be recorded.
- The data might not be reliably recorded.

Recording Critical (Significant) Incidents

Critical Incident Analysis – also known as Significant Incident Analysis – is also used within action research, to complement and supplement other forms of data. A Critical or Significant Incident Log can also be used as an effective tool for critical reflection. Recording events and analysing the accounts for meanings can offer insights into changing aspects of practice. It is advisable for all the research participants to be involved in recording these incidents. The log will include a snapshot of an event which is of relevance to the objectives of the study. These logs will then provide a common set of data from which learning and theory making can follow. Hills et al. (2007) report the use of a modified critical incident technique where care team members were asked to recall incidents when key elements were effectively implemented during interviews, throughout which reflection was encouraged.

Advantages to recording Critical Incidents

- Provides context specific, rich, first-hand data.
- The records can form the basis for reflective discussions.
- It is possible to gather different perspectives from research participants.
- Recording significant incidents within an action research project can be very motivating and can also contribute to personal learning.
- Helps to stay focused on the aims of the project.

Possible disadvantages to recording Critical Incidents

- The choice of what to record may be challenging.
- There may be a temptation not to record sensitive issues and events.
- There is a possibility of misunderstanding, misinterpreting, and misrecording.
- There may be insufficient information recorded.
- Recorded incidents may be too descriptive and not useful at the time of analysis.

Quality indicators

Action research is a unique approach to carrying out enquiries into aspects of practice but the action researcher still needs to consider questions of validity, reliability, and generalisability within the context of the particular research study. In Chapter 6 we shall discuss these in greater detail.

First, we need to consider the *validity* of the data. This means we need to examine the accuracy of what is collected and used as evidence. We need to be aware that the conclusions are based on the quality of what we gather as data. Sometimes interpretations of the same event or evidence can vary between different people. This is due to their differing personal and professional life experiences. An awareness of how researchers have affected a project (reflexivity) is important in order to understand the process and outcomes of a study. This can affect the validity of the data presented.

Another way of establishing validity, according to Mason (2002: 246), is to find 'various means of confirmation, such as arranging for a colleague to observe as well, arranging for audio or video recordings, and asking other participants for their versions'. Mason recommends triangulation for this purpose, which he describes as the process of obtaining several viewpoints or perspectives. The word *triangulation,* he explains, is based on the method of surveying land which breaks the region down into triangles, each of which is measured. Hopkins (2002: 133) also emphasizes the role of triangulation in data-gathering, 'as it involves contrasting perceptions of one actor in a specific situation against other actors in the same situation. By doing so, an initial subjective observation or perception is fleshed out and gives a degree of authenticity'. In action research, different sources of data – field diaries, interview transcripts, questionnaire responses and observations, for example – can be put together to achieve a deeper and wider picture. In their review of action research projects. Waterman et al. (2001) found that in some studies there was recognition of the value of feeding back information to participants and discussing mechanics and purpose of this feedback. Feedback was viewed as an important stage of the action research cycle so that people could critically reflect on the findings to establish the next planning or replanning phase.

In the context of action research we also need to consider the aspect of *reliability.* Reliability is described as the consistency or stability of a measure (Robson, 2002) and a consideration of whether, if the measure were repeated, one would obtain the same result. If action researchers use a structured data collection tool, such as a questionnaire, they need to be reassured that it is reliable and valid. He maintains that, in general, most action researchers and those who use qualitative methods are concerned with validity rather than reliability, in so far as their focus is a particular case rather than a sample.

In the case of action research, the researcher needs to emphasize that generalizability is still possible, in terms of the project being applicable to other similar situations.

We would now wish to present a *practical task* for the reader to plan data gathering for a particular example of an action research project. Study the following scenario and consider what data will need to be collected to achieve the aims of the project.

Working title for the project: An action research project to increase the participation of women in the treatment and control of their diabetes

This project is being set up by four general practices, collaboratively, to encourage diabetes patients to attend surgery sessions regularly for check-ups and to adopt a greater engagement with treatment guidelines. The project is being initiated by one surgery where practitioners have noticed that a specific group of patients – i.e. South Asian women – did not keep their diabetic monitoring appointments, although reminders were sent out to them. It was also found that in the test for blood sugar control (HbA1c) the same group of women showed a lack of control compared to other patients. When this was mentioned in a meeting, which was attended by the practice representatives from other surgeries, it became clear that the problem was similar in three of the other surgeries. The project is being set up by the nursing staff in the four institutions, supported by one general practitioner in each surgery. One of the four general practitioners holds a part-time research position in a higher education institution and has volunteered to facilitate the research process if required. The project is set against the backdrop of UK healthcare policies which actively encourage practitioners to work with users and other agencies. The researchers have decided on three objectives for the project which is to run over 18 months.

- An exploration stage, in order to find out why attendance was low amongst this specific group.
- Seeking ways of encouraging attendance and planning activities to enhance patient understanding and participation.
- Evaluating the process and outcomes.

Summary

This chapter directed the reader's attention to all aspects of data collection within action research. Methodological issues were discussed extensively. Specific issues relating to the major paradigms used within action research were explored. The importance of addressing ethical issues was stressed and practical advice given. Extensive guidance on the different methods of data-gathering used within action research, and their relative merits and limitations, were discussed and these were supported by practical examples. Issues of validity, reliability, and generalizability, within the context of action research, were discussed and the role of triangulation as a means of quality control was also raised.

Further reading

Bell, J. (1999) *Doing your Research Project.* Buckingham: Open University Press.

Cohen, L., Manion, L. and Morrison, K. (2007) *Research Methods in Education* (6th edition). London: RoutledgeFalmer.

Creswell, J.W. (2009) *Research Design : Qualitative, Quantitative, and Mixed Methods Approaches.* Thousand Oaks, CA: SAGE.

Drever, E. (1995) *Using Semi-structured Interviews in Small-scale Research: A Teacher's Guide.* Edinburgh: SCRE.

Kvale, S. and Brinkman, S. (2009) *Interviews: Learning the Craft of Qualitative Research Interviewing.* London: SAGE.

Silverman, D. (2004) *Doing Qualitative Research: A Practical Handbook* (2nd edition). London: SAGE.

Stringer, E.T. and Genat, W.J. (2004) *Action Research in Health.* Upper Saddle River, NJ: Pearson Prentice-Hall.

Waterman, H., Tillen, D., Dickson, R. and de Koning, K. (2001) 'Action research: a systematic review and assessment for guidance', *Health Technology Assessment 5* (23).

6

Analysing data and generating evidence

This chapter focuses on:

- Organizing, analysing, and representing data
- A range of examples of data analysis
- The role of computer software in data analysis
- Validating evidence
- Making claims and contributing to knowledge.

Introduction

Imagine an action research project is now entering a crucial stage. It has been planned with meticulous attention and data have been gathered using different methods. Now it is time for the final analysis to be carried out and the data presented, prior to conclusions being drawn and the findings being shared. During this action research project, with its cycle of phases, researchers will have been making some form of analysis of the data and now, at this final stage, they will be pulling together all the findings, reflecting on their implications for practice, as well as identifying unanswered questions and new directions. The time it takes to analyse and present the data may depend on the nature of the project. For example, for a researcher who is undertaking a study which will lead to an academic dissertation, the process of analysis may take longer as there would be a larger amount of data to organize and analyse. Many of our students experience mixed feelings at the analysis stage. After many months of work, they may feel quite excited about the final analysis before drawing conclusions as this marks a significant stage in their research process, but they may also feel quite overwhelmed by the amount of data they have collected. We think if the data has been collected carefully and issues of validity have been addressed as researchers progressed through the study, the analysis stage should not pose any real difficulties.

As action researchers, we have to create a coherent and credible story from all the data collected. Researchers may have used a mixed methodology and collected some quantitative and qualitative data, but it is more likely that most of your data will be qualitative. We personally feel that analysing qualitative data is just as challenging as analysing and presenting quantitative evidence. At this point, action researchers also need to be aware of some of the criticisms made by many that action research is a 'soft' option in which the practitioner researcher works with a small number of people and therefore this is not 'proper' research. To address this criticism, were it warranted as not all action research is small scale, we would just reiterate what we have said previously – that an action researcher is involved in investigating a question or a topic within his or her own context and the focus will be on a single case or that of a small group of people. It may be part of the professional and personal development of those involved. An action researcher is looking to create meanings using rich descriptions and narratives. An action researcher develops expertise through looking at situations closely and analysing them, recognizing any possible bias and interpreting data, rather than looking to generalize the findings based on a study of large numbers of cases.

Making a start

Before starting the final stage of data analysis, it is important for action researchers to revisit the aims and expectations of a project. They must think about the research question and remind themselves of what it is they have been investigating. We suggest to our students that they write this out on a card and place it in a prominent position while they are working with the data. During data analysis researchers are trying to identify themes and patterns in order to be able to present robust evidence for any claims they are about to make. They need to look at the data they have collected from several sources and relate these to what were the original, expected outcomes. Of course, any good researcher would also be looking out for unexpected outcomes which may be of significance to report on these as well. The conclusions must also relate to the original aims and objectives or research questions of a project. It is also useful for researchers to remind themselves of reading all the literature they have accessed during a project, which should help with the analysis.

At this stage of the research, it is important for action researchers to reflect on the research process – from the initial stage of planning – and to make notes on how the proposed plan worked and about their experiences during data collection. It is possible that most of their ideas and organization went according to plan, but they may also have encountered unexpected problems and had to solve them. As we have discussed in earlier chapters, even after every best effort to make everything work out smoothly things can still go wrong, as in healthcare establishments unexpected challenges do occur. Anyone who would be interested in reading about the research and transferring the findings to their own settings would certainly also be interested in knowing about the difficulties experienced as well as the successes.

Organizing the data

Although it may sound obvious, here is a useful suggestion for any fledgling action researcher. As the researcher collects the data, he or she should make a note of all those collected and the numbers involved and from whom: for example, the number of questionnaires used; how many were sent and received back; how many interviews were conducted; who with and the length of each interview; how many people refused to be interviewed or observed and why; how many sessions were observed; who and what was observed and how many diaries have been kept; who they were given to and what they were asked to write about. This helps to keep the focus on all the datasets. When reporting the findings the researcher may wish to present these in a table (see the example in Table 6.1), which will provide the reader with an overview of the whole data-gathering exercise and a clear picture of all the datasets.

The next step is to have a look at the notes or personal journal that have been kept during data collection. The researcher may have been making some analysis of the data while it was being collected, this might include formal data analysis running parallel with data collection or personal notes on themes, which relate to the original research aims and questions. As this was being done the researcher may have made decisions about whether additional data was needed; this should be noted too. The researcher may also have been making a note of unanticipated themes or ideas emerging and spotted some shortcomings in the data collection methods. It is useful to remember these before starting on the final stage of data analysis and reporting.

In order to get started on a discussion of issues relating to data analysis, we have included examples of action research projects in the following section. These were carried out in several contexts and the time frame in which these happened varied from two to three years. These examples

TABLE 6.1 *Details of data collection*

Type of data	Who/what?	How was it collected?	How many?	Dates of collection
Questionnaires	45 staff nurses and 15 house officers working on five surgical wards	On-line	60 sent, 22 returned	16 September– 30 September
Interviews	Adult patients admitted as day cases for surgery	One-to-one semi-structured interviews	20 approached, 2 refused	1 October– 31 December
Observations	Interactions about the management of pain between patients and staff on surgical wards	Participant observation	180 hours spread over 1 month (60 hours 8am–12pm; 60 hours 12pm–8pm; 60 hours 8pm–8am)	2 January– 31 January
Diary	Personal reflections, analytical ideas, and reflexive commentary	Recorded onto personal computer	N/A	Throughout the project

should provide us with some reference points and help us to consider choices in selecting appropriate ways of analysing and presenting data.

Analysis and presentation of the data

Let us now consider some general issues about how a researcher would analyse and present the data. Before we start, we would need to consider the overall presentation of the article or report. By this we mean researchers would need to think about how the parts will fit into the whole so each section is linked to the whole document. One way of going about this would be to consider the purpose of each part and if/how it contributes to the overall article. If one element does not really add to the article, it is probably redundant.

Having thought about the overall purpose and presentation, it would be time to work on the analysis. As we mentioned earlier, it is likely that some quantifiable data has been collected alongside the qualitative data (as is the case in each of our examples that follow), but in many cases all the data collected may be qualitative – in the form of interviews, field notes, and researchers' diary entries.

Working with quantitative data

In action research a researcher may have collected some quantitative data which might help to supplement and complement the qualitative data collected. In action research projects, which are located within a professional situation and practice (which often forms part of a Master's or professional doctoral work), it is unlikely a massive amount of quantitative data will have been collected. Researchers should be able to analyse and represent the quantitative data using frequency counts which they can represent in tables or using charts. A computer package such as Excel is suitable for this purpose. If an action research project involves several sites and the data are extensive, a statistical package such as SPSS (http://SPSS.com) is worth considering. Support on using this package would be given on a research training course. A selection of useful reference books is provided at the end of this chapter.

Including charts and diagrams is helpful for two reasons. First, a visual display makes it easier for the reader to understand information. Secondly, these can break up continuous prose which can sometimes be tedious for a reader who is trying to make sense of numerical data. In a research project which explores the type of interactions that occur when patients request pain relief following surgery, a researcher may present such information as a frequency table which is easy to understand. This type of information can also be presented in graphical form. When data are displayed in this way, it is important for action researchers to remember not to emphasize the findings in percentage terms as they are only studying small numbers. Making claims in percentage terms does not create much impact when only referring to a total number of ten or twenty!

Another simple bit of advice we would extend here is that whatever the method you have chosen to analyze and display data, the story must be told effectively. Graphs and charts can look quite impressive, especially when in colour, but researchers should try to avoid displaying the same information twice (for example, both in a table form and through a number of colourful bar charts which just repeat the same information in a visual format). However, using tables is a simple and effective way to communicate findings. As in the earlier example in Table 6.1, making sure clear titles are provided, labelling each column, and giving a clear indication of the total numbers involved and what the headings mean are all advisable. It is often useful to ask colleagues (preferably those who have not been involved in the project) to look at tables to see if they can make sense of these in order to make adjustments as necessary.

It can be tempting in action research to collect data before and after an intervention to observe whether the second set of results is better than the first. While this has some merit (as it indicates what may happen in a full blown randomized controlled trial) the design is weak and will be criticized for being open to all sorts of confounding variables which could be responsible for the observed changes and not the intervention. Action researchers need to avoid making unwarranted claims for the effectiveness of their actions.

Action research is commonly employed to develop something, be it a new way of organizing a clinic or a healthcare role or an educational package for patients or staff. Quite often there will be no previous research available on which to base the proposed development and the action research team will have to research the subject for themselves. For example, in an action research project, we developed (a) a Hyperemesis Impact of Symptoms (HIS) questionnaire to ascertain how women were affected by severe nausea and vomiting in pregnancy (*hyperemesis gravidarum*) and (b) a prompt card which gave suggestions on how to give individualized care for women with this condition. In this action research project, we not only carried out qualitative semi-structured interviews with women to understand better about their experiences of severe nausea and vomiting in pregnancy, we also tested the questionnaire for its validity and reliability against other similar validated and reliable questionnaires, including a generic quality of life questionnaire and a severity of vomiting questionnaire. We compared scores from women with and without the condition to see if it would discriminate between the two groups. Figure 6.1 shows the difference visually (note that the higher the score the more severe the nausea and vomiting). In Figure 6.2, the bar graph shows visually that there

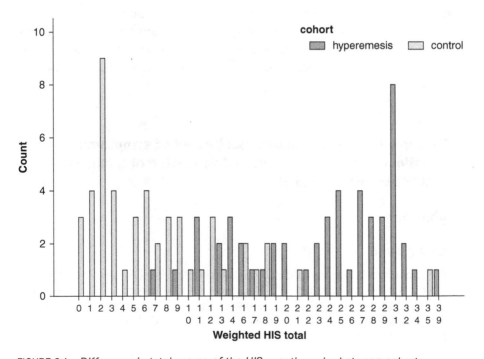

FIGURE 6.1   *Difference in total scores of the HIS questionnaire between cohorts*

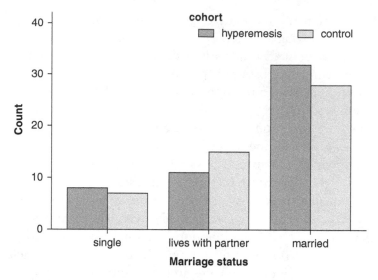

FIGURE 6.2   *Marital status of both groups*

was no significant difference in marital status between women with and without the condition.

The abstract from the published article from this aspect of the action research can be found below. The abstract gives an idea of the statistical testing which we carried out to show that the questionnaire was valid and reliable. In this instance we felt that given the amount and quality of the data on the validation of the questionnaire this warranted publishing these in their own right even though these were developed in an action research project.

Example 6.1   The hyperemesis impact of symptoms questionnaire: development and validation of a clinical tool (Power et al., 2010)

Abstract

Background

The Hyperemesis Impact of Symptoms Questionnaire is a clinical tool designed to assess holistically the impact of the physical and psychosocial symptoms of hyperemesisgravidarum (HG) on individuals. Its purpose is to aid the planning and implementation of tailored care for women with HG. To our knowledge no similar tool exists.

Objective

To assess the validity and reliability of the HIS questionnaire.

Design

As no similar tool exists, we compared the HIS with three tools that reflected its key areas: physical impact (Pregnancy Unique Quantification of Emesis – PUQE score and markers of severity of HG), psychological impact (Hospital Anxiety and Depression Score – HADS), and social impact (SF12 quality of life score).

Setting

A large regional referral, women, and children's hospital in the North West of England.

Participants

The HIS was evaluated on 50 women admitted to hospital with HG and 50 women recruited from an ante-natal clinic without severe nausea and vomiting and with an uncomplicated pregnancy.

Results

Good criterion validity was demonstrated by strong significant correlations with all three scores (PUQE, $r = 0.75$, $p < 0.001$, HADS, depression $r = 0.76$, $p < 0.001$, and SF12, mental component $r = \_0.65$, $p < 0.001$). The HIS showed good internal consistency, Cronbach alpha 0.87, split half 0.80.

Conclusions

There is evidence for the validity and reliability of the HIS to assess the impact of the physical and psychosocial symptoms of HG. Further research is currently underway to establish the clinical utility of the HIS questionnaire in the care of women hospitalized with HG.

Not all action research projects will require such statistical skills but should a researcher require more complicated statistics they must not hesitate to locate a statistician who can help.

Working with qualitative data

As action research is usually located within a professional context and practice, researchers would be exploring attitudes, behaviour and feelings which would necessitate the gathering of qualitative data that they will need to analyse and interpret. The data collected are likely to include open-ended questionnaires, interviews, observation notes, personal logs and so on, most of which will be in the form of descriptive text. In the case of qualitative data, analysis of the text involves researchers making an analytical framework which can often be subjective so this needs careful addressing in terms of validity. If there is a large volume of text, the task of analysing all this can seem daunting, but the positive angle to this is that in an action research project the qualitative data from various sources will help researchers in gaining insights into the social reality of situations through the interpretations they make. If there is a considerable amount of descriptive data, one option is to use a computer package which is relatively simple to operate, as outlined later in this chapter. As a thorough account of computer packages is beyond the scope of this book, the reader is directed to the further reading at the end of this chapter.

Analysing qualitative data

There is no one correct way to analyse qualitative data, but one important factor that makes all data analysis effective is the need to be systematic. As we mentioned earlier, the data analysis may have started when researchers organized and carried out the data collection. The type of questions asked, the framework used for observations, and the nature of the documents collected would have been structured in such a way that researchers used various themes and categories as part of this process. A step-by-step approach we usually suggest to our students is as follows:

- Organize the data, listing the different sets collected.
- Read the content. This is to get a general feel of what the data are saying and how this relates to the original aim. All the data – observation notes, field diaries, policy documents and so on – will need to be looked at. Common words and themes should start to emerge.
- Highlight sections in the data which are relevant to the research area.
- If there is a range of data to analyse, generate codes for analysis. Coding is dealt with in later sections of this chapter.
- Construct categories from the codes to gather evidence. When reporting on findings use actual evidence (actual quotes, artifacts, etc.) from the data to back up any claims.
- Review the coded documents and categories and select any significant themes to report on.
- Interpret the findings.
- Write the report and plan the dissemination.

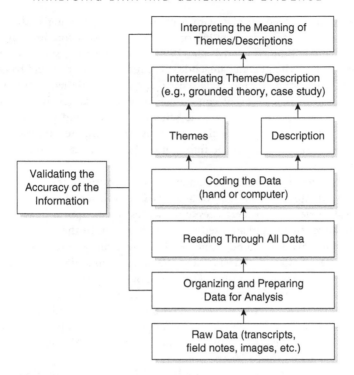

FIGURE 6.3   *Data Analysis in Qualitative Research (Creswell, 2009: 185)*

A framework for qualitative data analysis and interpretation

If a significant amount of qualitative data has been collected, Creswell's (2009) framework for qualitative data analysis and interpretation can prove a very useful guide (see Figure 6.3). Creswell points out that 'preparing the data for analysis, conducting different analyses and moving deeper and deeper into understanding' is like 'peeling back the layers of an onion' for qualitative researchers.

The step-by-step approach proposed by Creswell provides a very useful guide for practitioners undertaking action research. This is summarized for the reader in the following section.

- *Step 1* Organize and prepare the data for analysis. This involves transcribing interviews, scanning material, typing up notes, and sorting and arranging different types of data.
- *Step 2* Read through all the data. A first step is to obtain a general sense of the sets of information and to reflect on their overall meaning to gain a first impression, from the ideas and the tone of the ideas about the overall depth, credibility, and the use of the information. Researchers should make notes in the margin and record any general thoughts at this stage.

- *Step 3* Begin detailed analysis with a coding process. Coding is the process of organizing the material into chunks or segments of text before bringing meaning to information (Rossman and Rallis, 1998). Creswell's suggestions to researchers on what to use when coding are: code what readers expect to find based on past literature and common sense; code what is surprising and unanticipated; code for the unusual which may be of conceptual interest to readers. Researchers could hand-code the data, use colour code schemes, and cut and paste text segments onto cards. The other option at this stage is using a computer software package to help code, organize, and sort the information (see the next section for the use of computer software).
- *Step 4* Use the coding process to generate a description of the setting or people, as well as categories of themes for analysis. Creswell suggests generating five to seven categories. These categories and themes would appear as major findings in qualitative studies and are used to create headings in the findings sections of studies. These would also be supported by quotations and specific evidence.
- *Step 5* Researchers should decide how the description and themes will be represented in the qualitative narrative. The most popular approach is to use a narrative passage to convey the findings of the analysis. This might be a discussion that mentions a chronology of events, the detailed discussion of several themes (complete with sub-themes, specific illustrations, multiple perspectives from individuals, and quotations), or a discussion with interconnecting themes. Visuals, figures, or tables as adjuncts may be used with the discussion.
- *Step 6* This final step involves researchers making an interpretation or deriving meaning for the data. Questions about what lessons have been learnt must be asked. These lessons would be based on researchers' interpretations. These may also take into account any information gleaned from the literature or theories that confirm or diverge from it and suggesting new questions which may not have been foreseen earlier in the study.

Reflexivity and qualitative data

The issue of reflexivity needs to be considered when reporting on findings, as a researcher's own social identity and background will impact on the research process. As previously discussed, reflexivity is an important component of demonstrating the validity of a project. For example, reflexivity is important for a healthcare action researcher who is planning and implementing the action in a healthcare setting while they are also a practitioner. In such circumstances, this researcher would need to reflect on the possible impact of being a practitioner-researcher and acknowledge the possible influence this may have on the interpretations they make and the bias which may influence the research process. As Creswell (2009: 177) points out, qualitative research is interpretive research with the inquirer typically involved in a sustained and intensive experience with the participants which 'introduces a range of strategic, ethical and personal issues into the qualitative research process' (Locke et al., 2007).

Strengths of qualitative data within action research

As a final reflection on the use of qualitative data, we would stress that qualitative data have some particular strengths for the action researcher. In a very illuminating textbook focusing on qualitative data analysis, Miles and Huberman (1994: 10) indicate the features of qualitative data which contribute to its strength as 'its focus on naturally occurring, ordinary events in natural settings, so that we have a strong handle on what "real life" is like'. The authors describe the quality of its 'local groundness', as the data are collected in close proximity to a specific situation. What also makes qualitative data very suitable for the action researcher, according to the authors, is the fact that such data can capture the 'richness' and 'holism' of a situation.

Other forms of data analysis

Some action researchers will use the *constant comparative method,* a principle used within *grounded theory* (Glaser and Strauss, 1967; Strauss and Corbin, 1998) for data analysis. This involves researchers comparing data from all the sources – interviews, observations and documentation. Detailed and systematic coding is undertaken and categories are formed. Differences and similarities within categories are then established while theory is developed from grounded data. This is a lengthy, but a very established process, used by action researchers as reported in studies within healthcare. Another method used within action research is *content analysis*, a process by which 'the many words of the text are classified into much fewer categories. (Webber, 1990: 15). Content analysis can be undertaken with any written material, such as interview transcripts, documentary evidence, open-ended questionnaire responses, or personal notes, but quite often this method of analysis will be used when there is a large amount of data to be categorized.

Using computer software for data analysis

Using computer software for analysing qualitative data is another option available to action researchers. However, as Mertler (2006) points out, it is a misconception to think that the software will do the analysis as data analysis still needs the use of inductive logic which can only occur in the human brain. The author reminds us that even advanced technologies cannot take the place of human logic. What computer packages can effectively do is help researchers to store and organize the data if these are typed up. They can also provide a system for coding and categorizing the data from all the notes and transcripts electronically, thus enabling researchers to search for key phrases and words. However, if this were a project which involved collecting a large amount of qualitative data, using computer packages may be a good option. Most universities will provide both access to such packages and training on how to use these.

Coding

One means of organizing and understanding data is to code the text. Coding is simply identifying the main themes and patterns within data. Its purpose is for researchers to conceptualize and reduce the data (Strauss and Corbin, 1998) to fit into a manageable format from which to make conclusions.

There are many ways to code. Whatever the method chosen, the most important things to bear in mind are research questions and research aims. After transcribing all of the interviews, or immersing themselves in any other data sources, it is highly likely researchers will feel overwhelmed. There are two main feelings about the data to battle with. Firstly, there may be a feeling that all of the data are important and relevant, which can consequently lead to a panic about leaving something out (Auerbach and Silverstein, 2003). Coding should reduce this worry, as once researchers begin to look for similar themes and patterns, the data will feel much more manageable and it will become clearer what the relevant issues are. It is likely researchers will feel all data are interesting but, again, it is important to remember the research questions and aims; if the data are not relevant to the aims, they are not relevant to researchers currently but may raise new questions and suggest future directions for their research. Once they begin to realize they are only coding things which are relevant, they will begin to feel in control of the datasets.

Coding can be hard work, but the tedium of doing so can be overcome by adopting techniques similar to those used when revising for tests! Regular breaks should be taken, in order to maintain full concentration, as well as frequently reviewing the coding criteria.

Many forms of data can be coded, although the most common is interview transcripts. It is also possible to code the open-ended responses to questionnaire and survey results, as is the case with more closed ended questions.

Example of coding for analysing an interview

Below is a typical excerpt from a transcribed interview with a patient with glaucoma. The aim of this action research was to find out whether and why patients choose to adhere to their prescribed eye drops for glaucoma, whether they have specific educational needs and preferences, and to develop and evaluate a group-based educational programme for patients on glaucoma treatment. In the right-hand column are sequential quotes from the interview. In the left-hand column, are broad themes in italics beneath which are codes. The reader will note that the reason for this patient's non-attendance at clinic was that there was no confirmation of a diagnosis. Non-adherence to glaucoma eye drops was because of lack of knowledge of (1) the need for renewal of prescription and (2) that eye drops were for life. This kind of information would be useful in knowing what to include in an educational programme for patients.

Adherence to eye drops Type: Unclear diagnosis Not attending appointments	Q: Um, so you … just tell me, have you been diagnosed with glaucoma now? A: Yes. Q: You have? A: Umm, it was 'bout 15 years ago when I went to the optician for an eye test when it was first spotted, I think. Q: Hmmmm. A: And she sent me for a field (test) … at the hospital, then after that they were undecided, yes it was, then no it wasn't, yes it was, no it wasn't, had this carry on for a few years. Then I didn't bother with going for appointments for a couple of years and then I thought I should go back for another eye test at the end of last year … Q: Hmmmm. A: … and she told me I needed to go back to the eye doctor. Q: Right.
Adherence to eye drops Type: Not attending appointments Reason: Felt they were doing nothing for him	A: So I had had a two year break from attending the eye hospital because it seemed that they were doing nothing for me when I went back after the break I saw another doctor. Q: Oh okay. A: That was when I was told it was definitely glaucoma and I was given eye drops. (voices overlap)

Adherence to eye drops	And how long ago was that that you started your drops?
Reason: Non-adherence due to misunderstanding about the drops	A: Oh started last February but I haven't been putting any in recently for the last few months … Q: Hmmmm. A: … I thought you put them in just the once and that would cure it. I was not told at that stage that they were for life I didn't know. I thought they were like anti-biotics which you take for a short period. Q: Ah … A: So I didn't put any in for about three months but after I went to the hospital, I learnt now that I need to get a repeat prescription from my doctor for them.
Adherence to eye drops Outcome: Feels he knows what to do now	Q: Okay. A So I think I am on top of it now.

Qualitative data can also be analysed to develop items for questionnaires. We did this in the action research project with women with severe nausea and vomiting in pregnancy. Table 6.2 shows the questions which were developed from some of the raw data.

TABLE 6.2 *Example evidence supporting the formulation of questions for the HIS questionnaire*

HIS Question	Examples of interview evidence to support question formulation
1 Are you able to keep small drinks down without vomiting?	*"You think maybe it is just going to be the morning, a one-off, but then suddenly you know it is twice in an hour and then it is retching and then you just can't stop."* *"I felt that I was dying. I was completely dry, I couldn't even sip water, I couldn't even swallow, I had no saliva."*
2 Are you able to keep small amounts of food down without vomiting?	*"Anything I've eaten since Sunday has just been coming out. So yesterday, all day, I just didn't eat anything. You're starving as well, which is funny, because you want to eat as well, but you can't keep it in."*
3 How tired do you feel?	*"I was woken up feeling sick, I couldn't get to sleep, because I was getting up every ten/fifteen minutes feeling sick. It was all through the day so I wasn't sleeping properly... I couldn't talk I didn't have no energy"* *"Just to have a bath or a shower would take so much energy up and I would just think no I can't, I can't – just to get out of bed."*

TABLE 6.2 *(Continued)*

HIS Question	Examples of interview evidence to support question formulation
4 Think back to your usual mood/emotional state before you felt sick, how do you feel now in comparison?	*"But it is the most miserable thing I've ever had because I've never really been ill before."* *"Very depressed because the main thing depressing was not the baby, it's the work. Mainly because if I take off sick, people won't be happy at all at work."*
5 Do you worry about the health of your unborn baby?	*"The main thing on your mind when you are not eating, is the baby not eating."* *"I was quite worried during that time about my baby, even though it wasn't my fault, I was trying to eat something, but I couldn't eat anything."*
6 Do you feel defeated by your nausea and vomiting and that nothing will work to make you feel better?	*"Nothing, no anti-sickness, no anti-emetics, nothing helped at all...We tried everything, but nothing helped."*
7 Do your symptoms effect your ability to look after your home and/or family?	*"This is taking over my life and I am not able to look after my son at the moment without help of other members of family and its unfair on him as he is unable to understand and he gets upset 'cos he knows I'm not well so he is extra clingy you know, if I'm not well I want to be just left alone but obviously at the same time I want to be able to care for him and play with him and everything, which at the moment I am not able to do."* *Researcher – Your little girl she's on holiday at the moment, how do you manage with that?* *"I couldn't, my Mum's got her. I couldn't cope. I couldn't even get her dressed, I couldn't even get me up and about, so I couldn't look after *****. I couldn't."*
8 Do you feel people understand how ill you are feeling?	*"It was like he wouldn't believe what I'm saying, that I've been sick and everything, literally. He was just like, nothing's wrong with you and I was like..., that day I was so bad, I couldn't even talk properly, so I felt a bit terrible."* *"I felt dismissed many, many times."*
9 Do your symptoms affect your worklife?	*"I haven't been able to go to work. I tried a couple of times in the last two weeks and had to come back early."* *"Even when the vomiting stopped, I could not return to work as I felt dizzy."*
10 Do your symptoms effect your ability to look after yourself?	*"You can't do anything yourself; totally depending on others, especially my husband. I couldn't even stand up myself last time; even to go to the toilet I had my husband's help. I had no strength at all even to get up."* *"Sometimes just going up the stairs to have a bath drains you so very much, so completely. By the time I get back downstairs, my legs are shaking."*

Source: Power, Z., Campbell, M., Kilcoyne, P., Kitchener, H. and Waterman, H. (2010) 'The Hyperemesis Impact of Symptoms Questionnaire: development and validation of a clinical tool', *International Journal of Nursing Studies*, 47: 67–77.

Computer Aided Qualitative Data Analysis Software (CAQDAS)

Computer software for aiding the qualitative textual analysis process has long been around, but it is only in the last two decades that researchers have begun to realize its full potential and make it a part of the normal research process. During the 1980s a wide range of packages was developed and today there still remain over 20 to choose from. Traditional coding used very simple and traditional tools, pencils, and coloured highlighters. The introduction of CAQDAS has brought transparency and discipline into qualitative analysis (Gaskell, 2000). Kelle (2000) has written an illuminative chapter on computer-assisted analysis in Gaskell (2000).

As there are so many CAQDAS programs, this section can only mention those most commonly used and the ones which will be included within the training courses offered by universities. These are only brief guidelines on how these programs can assist you with your data analysis; there is a vast array of specialist books on the market which can provide more detailed step-by-step guides of how to use each program, some of which are listed at the end of this chapter.

NVivo

NVivo is the most recent textual analysis programme to be produced by QSR, who made a name for themselves with the programme NUD*IST which was developed in the 1980s and has been developing ever since (Bazeley, 2007). To our knowledge NVivo is the most widely used qualitative textual analysis software, with several institutions running training courses on it, and is often taught on Master's programmes.

Atlas.ti

Atlas.ti is another computer-based software item which enables researchers to organize text, graphics, and audio and visual data files as well helping with text coding. It is important to note that the software does not do analysis for the researcher but helps to organise and display the data.

Using electronic reference management software

As mentioned in Chapter 3, it is worth remembering that several computer software packages exist which can help researchers to manage their references. Examples include EndNote, Procite, BiblioExpress and Reference Manager. Many of these can be used with word processing packages by directly importing references into the text. Some of these packages are free while others can be accessed through institutions or university libraries. It is worthwhile for researchers to invest the time to learn to use these software packages and, as always, working with someone who has used a package before can save time and avoid unnecessary frustrations. The initial investment of a few hours and a little effort is well worth it.

Using evidence and generating knowledge

When we discuss data analysis with our students, we start with the question 'Why do we gather data?' The main purpose of gathering data is to provide evidence. In order to provide evidence we need to analyse the data collected. Again, the starting point is to constantly remind oneself what one is really looking for. One can set out the aims at the start of the research and plan the data-gathering carefully, which has given a good starting point for gathering evidence to articulating the claims as well as for building personal theories.

Whether a researcher has collected quantitative data or qualitative data or a combination of the two, it is important to remember that ultimately the value of such research will depend on the quality of the type of data collected, the interpretations made, the personal reflections and conclusions. The significance of a project will depend on the way the data have been collected and analysed.

During data analysis, whether this is done manually or using a computer package, it will be useful for researchers to highlight parts which can be used as *evidence* when making claims and sharing research. With our students, we suggest that they colour-code different types of evidence under sections: how the original aims were met, what problems were encountered during the project in terms of practical day-to-day events, as well as any methodological aspects. The personal learning, implications, and practical significance of the research for researchers and others – as well as new questions and research directions – could also be noted. In the final report all of these aspects will need to be included.

So what do we mean by providing evidence? Take the previous example of the action research project in which we aimed to improve the care of patients who needed to lie face down for two weeks after retinal surgery. Patients found this post-operative instruction difficult to comply with and frequently did not persist with it. Initially the project aimed to understand why this was the case and gathered evidence using staff interviews and patient letters. This was compared to data from observations of the nursing care. From this the action research group decided, among other things, to set up pre-operative clinics to educate patients well in advance of the surgery about the post-operative requirements. Posturing equipment was bought and loaned to patients to help them lie face down at home. Educational sessions were also provided for staff to explain how and why patients should be encouraged to posture face down. Then further evidence was collected in the form of more patient letters and staff interviews to find out whether the initial issues had been resolved and to learn what further problems still existed. A qualitative evaluation provided us with important information on how people's understanding and practice had changed over time. It also produced unanticipated but nevertheless important outcomes for the research and their implications. For example, while we knew communication between staff was an important issue it was one of the hardest to tackle.

Generating knowledge

The purpose of research is to generate new knowledge and in an action researcher's case the knowledge produced is based on practice and all aspects of it – planning, what has been read, the data collection, action taken, evaluation of this, and what has been found out. Articulating the knowledge generated and how it has affected practice together with the significance it may have for other practitioners would be part of this. Researchers are building personal and group theories based on what they have done. The group theory arising from the example relating to the action research project to improve the care of patients who needed to posture face down after retinal surgery was that posturing was a shared responsibility between patients, nurses, and doctors. In other words, the focus should not be solely on the patients and blaming them when they do not comply. We learnt what were the social, demographic, communicative, and cognitive behavioural and emotional aspects to the issue and that for patients, nurses, and doctors these all played out slightly differently. For example, nurses had to demonstrate empathy with patients who were posturing, they needed to give patients the resources to posture, they needed to provide comfort to patients and to be their advocates when they could not do this for themselves.

Thus theories emerge from practice. A researcher contributes to knowledge and provides illustrative examples of what happened and quotes relevant evidence. The claims made and the theories formulated are original, as researchers have employed their own critical thinking and judgement skills. Remember that in order to make valid claims to knowledge, researchers will also have to back up their claims with evidence by using relevant parts of the data; this may consist of extracts from interview transcripts, selected sections from their notes of observation, artifacts, and photographs. One of our students included photographs of a relatively unknown piece of equipment that was important to his study so that readers could understand how it was situated in a ward setting.

Validating claims to knowledge

Research findings and claims to knowledge will be more powerful if researchers validate them. Action research is mostly carried out in collaborative teams involving action research groups, or Communities of Enquiry; this makes it easier to seek common understandings and interpretations so findings are more representative. The trustworthiness of research is also judged in terms of how the claims to knowledge are accepted by those who read the reports and published articles. So, how do researchers validate their claims to knowledge, bearing in mind readers will evaluate these critically. For the purpose of validation the first step is to articulate the procedures clearly, explaining how the research was conducted, how robust the methods of data collection were, and how triangulation (see Chapter 5) was achieved. Researchers should expect to be challenged in all aspects of the research claims they make. As previously highlighted, another important component of demonstrating the validity of work is being reflexive. A discussion of how researchers were reflexive and how their past experiences might have influenced how they have interpreted the data will be necessary.

We encourage our students to organize meetings with different groups of people who would consider their research processes and findings from different perspectives both during that research and at the conclusion of a project. For example, the first audience may be the action research group or fellow researchers during a seminar presentation. This may be less daunting, but the danger is that fellow researchers don't always ask harsh questions as they may have a particular empathy for researchers' situations and don't want to give them a 'hard time'. If a researcher is based in a healthcare centre, the audience could consist of colleagues (including those who were not part of the project) and audit teams. Inviting colleagues from healthcare establishments, especially those who have similar roles and responsibilities within their institutions, is also a good strategy. When reporting on research, a researcher must include details of the validity of their study.

Part of the role of the action research group is to challenge one anothers' assumptions; to present a balanced analysis of the study findings and process; to consider, critically, the ethical issues and the usefulness and transferability of the research. It is useful to circulate documents to independent but interested parties, academics, clinicians, and users, to read and comment individually and to give you formative feedback at different points of the research, as it is not necessary to have group meetings all the time. Writing up summaries of these meetings is useful in order to keep monitoring the quality of the action research, especially in order to check on the following aspects:

- Has the researcher focused on the research aims or questions?
- Are the action plans clear and realistic?
- Is the researcher aware of ethical considerations?
- Are the data collection and analysis procedures robust?
- Does the researcher have appropriate evidence for the claims they intend to make?
- Are they able to demonstrate critical awareness?
- Is the research likely to contribute to new knowledge?

Summary

This chapter focused on the data analysis which precedes the writing up of a report and the publication of findings. Various forms of data summaries were presented. Using examples of action research projects involving practitioners, aspects of organizing, analysing, and representing data were addressed. A framework for qualitative data analysis was provided, along with a discussion of the extraction of themes and patterns emerging from the collected data. Issues of reflexivity were considered. The use of computer software in data analysis was briefly discussed. The chapter concluded with a discussion of the importance of using evidence and generating and validating knowledge before claims are made.

Further reading

Auerbach, C.F. and Silverstein, L.B. (2003) *Qualitative Data: An Introduction to Coding and Analysis.* New York: New York University Press.

Bazeley, P. (2007) *Qualitative Data Analysis with NVivo.* London: SAGE.

Creswell, J.W. (2009) *Research Design: Qualitative, Quantitative, and Mixed Methods Approaches.* Thousand Oaks, CA: SAGE.

Gaskell, G. (2000) 'Individual and group interviewing', in M.W. Bauer and G. Gaskell (eds), *Qualitative Researching with Text, Image and Sound.* London: SAGE.

Huberman, A. and Miles, M.B. (1998) 'Data management and analysis methods', in N. Denzin and Y. Lincoln (eds), *Collecting and Interpreting Qualitative Materials.* Thousand Oaks, CA: SAGE.

Kelle, U. (2000) 'Computer-assisted analysis: coding and indexing', in M.W. Bauer and G. Gaskell (eds), *Qualitative Researching with Text, Image and Sound.* London: SAGE.

Strauss, A. and Corbin, J. (1998) *Basics of Qualitative Research: Techniques and Procedures for Developing Grounded Theory.* Thousand Oaks, CA: SAGE.

7

Writing Up and Publishing Action Research

This chapter focuses on:

- The process of writing up action research
- The structure of dissertations
- Why researchers should disseminate the outcomes of action research
- The various ways to disseminate
- Publishing in professional circles
- Publishing in academic outlets.

Introduction

We will start this chapter with a quotation from one of our PhD students which captures the spirit of what we want to say in this chapter.

> The process of writing up my action research study allowed the fragmented journey I had encountered to emerge as a fluid whole. Decisions I made regarding the elements I thought necessary to recount and also about where they started and ended in the narrative were as much statements about myself and my values as they were about the study and this reflexive awareness grew along with the report.

> Throughout the writing-up process I gained powerful insights into my choices, motivations, and assumptions at different junctures of the research. These insights exposed personal and professional traits which permeated the account though only became evident retrospectively through my narration. The written account became a personal synthesis of the stories which could have been told and although the final version gave rise to as many questions as answers, it gave me a deeper understanding of how I'd interacted with the research to interpret meanings and shape the action.

Jodie, like many other practitioners, carried out an action research project on a topic which arose from her intrinsic motivation to improve her practice. She also selected this study for her PhD thesis. She found the whole process of writing her thesis a challenging but rewarding experience. Not all action researchers are expected to produce a thesis or even a written report, but for those who are in the process of writing a final report of their action research, dissertation or thesis, useful guidance will be provided in this chapter.

At this point, we will reflect on our own experiences as action researchers and in our role of supporting action researchers in a variety of contexts. After carrying out a study which may last for several months or for even years, depending on the circumstances, there comes a time when we must produce a written report for an institution or sponsor or for the purpose of obtaining a qualification.

Writing a report of action research

Whether writing a report as part of the requirements for an accredited course or for the purpose of just making it available for others to read, here are some factors for the reader to consider. The need to be clear about what kind of a report it is and that as action research it need not necessarily be presented in the same way as more conventional forms of research must be paramount. The mode of study selected was action research and the purpose of action research is to improve practice or to implement change as a result of research.

What kind of report?

From the outset, it is important to consider the audience, the requirements, and the purpose of the report.

Consider the audience
Ask who is my audience? Perhaps there has been funding from an external source for the research and, in such cases, there may have been a specific format to follow, but it is not unusual for guidance to be unforthcoming. In those situations the following headings may be useful:

- [Executive summary].
- Aims.
- Background.

- Method of the action research.
- Summary of findings.
- Conclusion.

It may be that the researcher is writing a report or dissertation as part of the requirement for a qualification. In this case, the resulting work will be read by academic tutors and sometimes by an external examiner. If this is its purpose the author will be expected to follow a particular format and the conventions of scholarship. In a long study or a dissertation they will also be expected to show knowledge of recent and relevant research literature. Whatever the purpose, it is important to be clear and consistent and to demonstrate a good understanding of the issues researched. In the case of a dissertation or thesis for accreditation purposes, the expectation will be that the study has been extensive as the author would be considering themself an expert in the chosen area for study. While reporting action research, the quality of the writing can be enhanced by writing in an authentic and personal style. We have always felt that reporting action research is often powerful for one's own professional development because of the personal nature of the writing. It is helpful to remember that in reporting on a study the researcher will have constructed this from their experiences and collaborations with other people.

Think of the reader

A useful strategy to adopt when writing a report is to consider any of the potential readers of it. The following guidance may be of help to researchers:

- Always provide the background to a study and the context as action researchers. This helps the reader to relate to the report and possibly apply the findings to their own circumstances.
- It is important to present the aims at the outset and also the findings within the context of what they set out to achieve.
- Readers appreciate realism and honesty. It makes sense to report what has progressed magnificently as well as any difficulties experienced.
- Present the plans and outlines of action clearly. It is possible that others may want to carry out a similar study, or implement similar changes to practice, or report the findings to their colleagues.
- As action research is often a personal journey, writing the report in the first person is more effective. Sentences such as 'I chose this method because I had the opportunity to study this as part of my professional development ... ' or 'I changed direction after finding out ... ' makes the text reader-friendly and more accessible.
- Don't assume that readers always know what a researcher is discussing. Try and explain all aspects of a study in simple, clear language. Keep the target audience in

mind. If the report is going to be read by patients and carers, it would be inadvisable to use medical jargon.

- Use sub-headings where possible. It is easier to read text if it contains sub-headings.
- Be creative in the presentation. This is possible within any given format. Some of our students have used bubbles, cartoons and photographs containing evidence, when they presented their findings but do bear your audience in mind.

Writing a Master's dissertation

In this section, we will try to provide some guidance on writing a dissertation based on action research. These are not, by any means, meant to be definitive guidelines. We do not believe that a fixed set of rules can ever be applicable when writing up action research, because at the very heart of an action research project is the opportunity to be flexible, emergent, and creative. However, if the reader is writing a dissertation for accreditation purposes, they will need to follow the format given by the institution. Within that set format, there will still be plenty of opportunities to be original.

A dissertation is the culmination of the work undertaken which should demonstrate to readers a researcher's understanding of an issue, any action that has been taken, and how these actions have informed and developed practice and a researcher's professional life. The emphasis may vary depending on the institution but it could be on what was found out and the personal learning, though researchers need to be wary of making generalized claims for their work.

As the study is likely to be an inquiry into local practice, researchers need to pay attention to the following:

- Acknowledge one's own beliefs, prior assumptions, and values within the report, at the start (see Chapters 1 and 6).
- Acknowledge one's inevitable subjectivity, up front.
- Say, at the outset, what makes the approach valid.
- State clearly what methods were used for data-gathering and how multiple perspectives were sought.
- Discuss any ethical issues and how these have been addressed.

Maintaining quality

If the reader has been given a set of criteria for grading a dissertation, they must read them first. The following general checklist should help them to monitor the quality of the work. Have they:

- made the aims and objectives clear?
- justified why they are undertaking the work – providing a rationale?
- acknowledged their own perspectives and beliefs?
- made the context clear (this is important as action research, in most cases, is located within a distinct situation)?
- demonstrated their understanding of issues relating to the topic?
- shown that they have made efforts to read work carried out by others in the area for research and any theoretical literature relating to the study?
- articulated how prior stages of the process informed the next?
- shown how the work was participatory?
- explained how the data were collected and how they were valid?
- presented the data in an accessible manner and in such a way that someone reading it can identify the evidence generated for the conclusions?
- made coherent arguments?
- demonstrated personal learning?
- made recommendations for practice, policy, and further research?

All dissertations should also demonstrate the following features:

- a clear formulation of the research question or topic of study;
- a *critical* account of theories and research, including personal viewpoints and commentary;
- justified methods of inquiry;
- clearly presented data;
- ethical procedures;
- a robust analysis of the data;
- generated knowledge based on evidence;
- a critical discussion of the findings and emerging issues;
- a reflection on both the findings and the methodology used;
- any limitations;
- an enhancement of personal knowledge;
- a reflection on personal action and future directions;
- an organized bibliography.

Structuring a dissertation

As mentioned previously, higher education institutions will usually provide a basic format for writing a dissertation. A close study of the formats issued by a few institutions showed that although there were differences in the words used to describe the different parts of a dissertation, they all seemed to require similar content. In the following section, we will present a set of guidelines. These are in the form of chapter headings for writing a dissertation. As guidance notes they may be adapted for all courses leading to a qualification. Remember that we are referring to the format of a dissertation which arises from carrying out an action research project.

Doctoral theses

If the reader is undertaking doctoral work, using an action research approach, the framework for a thesis may still be similar to that of a Master's dissertation, but a higher degree of critical engagement with the existing theory and literature and a greater depth and conceptual analysis will be expected. The reader will also need to articulate their philosophical and theoretical perspectives in greater detail and show how the work is original.

Abstract

This section will provide a short summary of the aims, methodology, findings, and implications for practice. This must be a *brief* section – about 200 words should be sufficient. Many students will finalise their abstract after writing up the rest of the dissertation: this is wise because during the writing-up process thoughts will come together and help present an effective abstract. Do remember that the abstract is the first section of a study read by a supervisor or examiner and first impressions are important. Don't forget a study may be placed in the library where others who are interested may read it. It is customary to use the past tense here, as the reader is reporting on what has already been done.

Table of contents
Chapter 1 – Introduction

This chapter sets the context for the study and discusses the reasons for undertaking it. What was the personal and professional motivation? Why at this time? What are the trends in the topic of study in terms of recent local, national, or international developments, using some references to the literature? What specific aspect of the topic is to be studied? If it is a research question this must be presented clearly. What are the aims? This chapter also provides a guide, in the form of signposts, for any reader about what to expect in each chapter; this needs to be in a short summarized form.

Chapter 2 – Review of the literature

This chapter should present a comprehensive review of the literature relating to the topic of study. References must be made to recent and relevant literature – policy, theory, and research – on the topic. Are there any current debates on the topic? What has been written about the topic and who were the authors? We often ask students to present the literature in themes. The ideas gathered from a literature search should be analysed. The purpose of this chapter is to locate the study within a framework informed by what is out there and what has already been discovered. This is, therefore, an important chapter which needs careful planning and organizing. Rather than listing each writer's views or theories, connecting different perspectives of different authors by drawing on similarities and contrasts in their thinking is preferable. Presenting a summary of what each author has said, without pulling the ideas together, makes for a tedious read. Use sub-headings where possible. Providing a critical commentary on what is being presented, including an assessment of the quality of the research, an overview of the strengths and limitations of the literature, and whether there any gaps in the literature, is worthwhile here.

Chapter 3 – Methodology

In a dissertation we need to acknowledge action research as the mode of study. State why action research was chosen. Discuss the features of action research which made it suitable for the study. Explain what action research is. State the epistemological and ontological stance briefly and explain how the methodology fits in with the philosophy adopted. Discuss very briefly how action research evolved, over the years, as a method of inquiry for practitioners. What models of action research are known about and what the understanding is of these models. What are the advantages of action research as a method? Relate these specifically to the project. Show the reader also an awareness of the limitations of action research and respond to these in terms of the study that is about to be embarked on. Say how and why an action research group was formed and how participation was maintained throughout the project.

Chapters 4 and 5

Chapters 4 and 5 will usually be presented as 'Method' and 'Results' respectively in conventional dissertations or theses. However, the process of action research may not lend itself to such a neat demarcation of events. Somehow the complexity of the action research process has to be conveyed in an understandable way. Our students in the past have overcome this problem in one of three ways.

First, they may choose to present the phases of their action research in chronological order: reflection, planning, action, and evaluation. They would discuss the aims and objectives of each phase and show how the preceding phase influenced the next. In this type of dissertation, it is possible for the phases to be presented as different chapters. In the Abstract of the PhD presented below the student had chronologically presented her work and shown her developing theoretical understanding of issues and how these informed the new in-service training for non-registered nurses to administer medicines.

Example 7.1   'Calculation of competence': factors affecting support worker role development (J.S. McCarthy, 2008 unpublished PhD, University of Manchester)

Abstract

The thesis details an action research study to develop the role of adult in-patient mental health support workers in an NHS Trust. The research questions sought to identify the contribution that support workers could make to local care provision and identify those factors which supported or inhibited a developed role. The relationship between competence and its utility in the workplace was also explored and the development of theory was pursued through the action research cycle.

The study involved two phases. The first phase used focus group interviews to gain an understanding of the existing support worker role and elicit perspectives regarding a developed role. The sample involved 16 individuals comprising support workers, nurses, and managers. The findings of the first phase indicated that support workers performed a communication and interpersonal function. Support workers' skill in relation to this function determined autonomy within their wider role as assessed by nurses undertaking an informal 'calculation of competence'. A preliminary theory was developed which informed the second phase.

After agreement was gained to develop a support worker role in relation to medication delivery, the second phase focused on the development of a training programme and the subsequent implementation and evaluation of the support worker medication role. Twelve individual interviews with nurses and support workers were conducted to evaluate the impact of the role in practice. The interview findings indicated that nurses granting consent was a key factor in determining whether support workers were able to enact the medication role. This appeared to be related to issues concerning perceived risk and protection. Meanwhile, perceptions regarding support worker aptitude emerged as a key influence for nurses when consenting to support workers undertaking activities.

Theoretical development culminated in the proposal of a conceptual model profiling the relationships between risk, consent, and autonomy as mediated by perceptions of protection and competence as being key influences on support worker utility. These concepts are new to the literature regarding support workers. The identification of their presence and influence individually and collectively presents an understanding of how they operate to both support and inhibit role development.

Second, students may prefer to present a shortened version of the whole process in one chapter and present all the findings together in a single chapter, especially when they intend to develop theory or use a theory to explain the findings. In the abstract presented below the authors used theory to frame a study on how to improve relationships between the carers for patients and staff who worked in nursing homes.

Example 7.2   Supporting relationships between family and staff in continuing care settings (Austin et al., 2009)

In this Canadian study, a participatory action research approach was used to examine the relationships between families of residents of traditional continuing care facilities and the health care team. The objectives were to (a) explore the formation and maintenance of family–staff relationships, with attention being paid to the relational elements of engagement and mutual respect; (b) explore family and staff perspectives of environmental supports and constraints; and (c) identify practical ways to support and enhance these relationships. Results indicate that the resource-constrained context of continuing care had directly impacted on family and staff relationships. The nature of these relationships is discussed using the themes of 'Everybody Knows Your Name', 'Loss and Laundry', 'It's the Little Things That Count', and 'The Chasm of Us Versus Them'. Families' and staff's ideas of behaviours that supported or undermined relationships were identified, as were concrete suggestions for improving family–staff relationships in traditional continuing care settings in Canada.

Third, when the project is very complex, one aspect of it may be presented. The abstract below, taken from an MPhil, is part of an action research project to improve the care of women with severe nausea and vomiting in pregnancy. The MPhil concentrated on the qualitative findings only.

Example 7. 3   The experience of *hyperemesis gravidarum* (Z. Power, unpublished MPhil, University of Manchester)

Abstract

Hyperemesis Gravidarum (HG) is a severe form of nausea and vomiting in pregnancy that is distressing, debilitating, and potentially life threatening. This thesis presents qualitative, exploratory data on the experience of HG from the

(Continued)

(Continued)

perspective of women with the condition and the healthcare professionals (hcps) caring for them. The study originated from difficulties identified by hcps managing HG in a hospital setting.

The purpose of the study was to provide data to inform the development and improvement of services for women with HG.

The overall methodology for the study was action research. Focus groups were used to collect data from the hcps, while individual interviews were used to collect data from the women with HG.

The over-riding theme that emerged from the data was that while showing some sympathy for women with HG, the majority of hcps associated negative feelings with caring for them. This finding was also reflected in the data of the women with HG, many of whom reported feeling dismissed and invalidated at times by some hcps.

In this thesis I propose that despite the generally caring approach of staff at the sample site women with HG are an unpopular patient group and, further-more, that amongst hcps, HG is stigmatised. Consequently, women are at times experiencing an element of prejudice which can result in suboptimal care. Evidence from the literature suggests that this phenomenon may not be limited to the sample site. The possible contributing factors to this situation are discussed.

The originality of this thesis lies in the examination of the unpopularity and stigmatisation of women with HG from the point of view of both hcps and women with the condition. To our knowledge such a study has not been con-ducted within the UK before.

Whatever the structure chosen, the aim must be to present a detailed account of what happened during a project and to present the findings fairly and effectively. These chapters should contain detailed narratives of what was done, highlighting the outcomes by using a range of techniques. Describe the design of the study and the preparations and planning that preceded action. Reveal how the project was participatory in accounts of the process. Justify the data collection methods and also show an awareness of the limitations of each method used. Make it clear how the data were analysed. State whether any of the action research group were involved in designing questionnaires, or carrying out and analysing interviews. Include evidence to back up any claims for changes made, for example, extracts from tape recordings, observations, and personal logs may be used. Documentary evidence can also be presented, for example, the minutes from meetings.

Show how the findings of the literature review and the data informed the changes to practice that were implemented. If action was revised, refer to the succession of action cycles within the action research. Avoid unwarranted claims. The findings presented in this chapter must inform the reader of the impact the project has made.

Ethical considerations should also be included. Justify how the issues of validity were addressed. Following the guidelines provided in Chapter 6 of this book may prove useful.

Chapter 6 – Discussion and Conclusions

Discuss the most important themes to have emerged from the study. Draw on other findings to show whether they reflect what others have found out. Discuss whether and why the study has generated evidence which contradicts the outcomes of studies carried out by others. Say what contribution the study has made to the body of literature as a whole, especially if it is original. Be clear about any conclusions. Give an account of any personal learning. Reflect on the outcomes of the project and think about the future direction of the study. State how the findings have influenced practice and discuss the implications of the research for practice and policy in general. The limitations of the work should also be discussed; this could include how parts of the study may have posed problems.

References
Appendices

Creative presentations of action research

Here we draw on our experiences of working with action researchers who have been creative in their presentation of findings. Some practitioners will present their research findings to colleagues and others at conferences before writing their final reports, as they believe that the preparation for the presentation can help bring their thoughts together. Others will present their research outcomes after writing up their reports. Some researchers will not actually write a formal report, but will choose to disseminate their research in other ways, which still serve the purpose of bringing their ideas together and reflecting on them before sharing their work with others. So what forms of presentations are possible? Here are some examples of how the researcher may present the outcomes of action research.

Poster displays

Penelope, a university lecturer in nursing, displayed the outcomes of her research on improving pain management for surgical patients, at an exhibition at the local hospital. Titles of the different sections of the poster were as follows:

Main title: Managing Ophthalmic and Oral and Maxillofacial Postoperative Pain

Subtitles:

- Study aim
- Introduction
- Method of inquiry
- Action research group
- Methods and sample
- Theoretical framework for analysis
- Findings
- Conclusions
- Acknowledgements.

The exhibition gave Penelope an opportunity to publicize her evidence and talk about it to others. With the rapid advancement of software packages these days, it is possible to create impressive displays.

Professional conference presentations

Another way of disseminating action research is for researchers to make presentations to interested audiences. Three examples of such presentations come to mind. One was a national presentation of a project by a research nurse which was exploring ways to improve the care of women who suffer from severe nausea and vomiting in pregnancy. Using PowerPoint slides she brought the project to life and generated a great deal of support and interest for the study which led to many of the multi-disciplinary participants sharing similar experiences.

The second presentation at a national conference involved two academics from a university working with a group of nurses who were co-presenters. The presentation was on how to help patients adhere to stringent post-operative instructions and required many strands of action. The presentation led to considerable interest among practitioners who wished to know more about how they could improve their practice and invitations to the co-presenters to come and talk to practitioners at other hospitals.

The third presentation of a project we have seen was a play written and presented by three mothers who had been closely involved in a local community project to improve access to health and social care services in a deprived area of a city in the United Kingdom. The play convincingly and effectively told the story of how their lives had been changed by taking part in the project.

Based on oral presentations we have attended, we have constructed a set of guidelines which may be of use to the reader:

- With a PowerPoint presentation, only include pointers on the slides and do not read from the slides; the audience will prefer to hear someone speak about their experiences. Keep eye contact at all times. It is a pleasure for others to see someone become animated whilst narrating their stories.
- Make the presentation interactive and depending on the time and purpose of talk, give the participants some short tasks which relate to the project. This keeps the interest and attention of the audience.
- Use examples whether about patients or situations. These may include short films and photographs which can act as documentaries.
- When presenting the evidence and outcomes, in addition to any charts and figures, show examples of patient care, extracts from interviews, and comments from evaluations.
- Don't assume that practitioners prefer not to know about the theories and research used in a project. Provide an overview of these that can give more academic and scholarly credibility. It is useful to give out a sample of readings and a set of references at the end of a presentation.
- Finally, give the audience an e-mail address to contact for further information if they wish. If visitors are acceptable, extend an invitation.

Academic research conferences

It is possible that the reader may wish to make a presentation at an academic research conference. The first step here is to look at the websites of research associations such as the Royal College of Nursing Research Society (http://www.rcn.org.uk/newsevents/news/article/uk/rcn_international_nursing_research_conference) or the Collaborative Action Research Network (http://research.edu.uea.ac.uk/links/care/collaborativeactionresearchnetworkuk). A few presentations on action research we have previously attended at the CARN conference have been from practising clinicians who were reporting research within their institutions and these sessions were well attended. The above websites will give information on the different formats of presentations to submit. For example, at both the conferences individual papers or poster presentations can be submitted. Some conferences have special support for novice presenters and these are worth enquiring after. In many cases a paper that has been accepted for presentation will prove suitable for publication in an academic journal.

Telling action research as a story

In recent times, stories of action research projects have been posted on websites. These stories are viewed as accessible to readers and one way to disseminate action research as they can offer a meaningful account to readers in a style that is suited to those who are interested in the practical implications of an action research project.

Writing an academic research report or article

So far, we have focused on writing up action research, with particular reference to writing dissertations. Now we shall explore the theme of sharing research with others more widely. Carrying out action research is an intrinsically satisfying activity. After much reading, planning and evaluating the research, the work is complete and it is time the new knowledge generated was shared with others. While carrying out research, it is highly likely that researchers will have been informally sharing experiences with colleagues in their institution and other professionals in the local area. If the research was funded by an external body, the funder will expect a report. If a research grant had been provided, the research funding body may expect researchers to disseminate their findings at research conferences and to write a few papers for publication in academic journals. We shall now offer more practical guidance on how to share findings in a range of ways both locally and globally.

Many of the practitioners we have worked with, on action research projects, have felt they don't have much to say to others. Sometimes they will feel writing is only for academics in universities and will lack the confidence to embark on this. During conversations with practitioners who have carried out action research, the following issues have been raised as acting as barriers to them publicizing their research.

'Surely it is doing the research which is important, not the writing'.

'No one is going to take note of what I have to say. I don't have the background or the expertise to publish'.

'Who will take note of what we, the nurses, have to say? No one will read it after all the effort'.

Whilst we would empathize with the misgivings and feelings of inadequacy felt by many, we have also shared the pleasure many of the practitioners feel when they do make conference presentations, contribute to a newsletter, publish their findings on a website, or publish papers in professional or academic journals.

So why do we think it is important to publicize action research? First, disseminating learning and what has been discovered are important for professional development. The process of writing up research and sharing it with other professionals and academics encourages the further construction of knowledge and reflection on ideas, reinforcing understanding and helping to ground ideas. Practitioners who have worked with us on action research projects have often felt a sense of worth and pride when they find out that their publications have been read by other professional colleagues. Then, of course, publishing research provides evidence of professional development and achievement and this addition to a *curriculum vitae* can often help towards promotions and progression in careers.

Publishing findings

Having decided to publicize their research more widely, the next question practioners will consider is how to go about making it a reality. Research can be communicated in various forms. In a newsletter for colleagues in the local area or in an institution's newsletter for patients and carers. Publishing research on a website is common these days; this can be an effective visual medium for presentation and may include an interactive element in it, so it will be possible to invite feedback and comments from other users. This contributes to on-going learning and the sharing of ideas, as this becomes part of a collaborative network of professionals and patients communicating ideas with each other. Research may also be communicated at national and international conferences or findings can be disseminated through a few of the above outlets. The various different forms of dissemination will require careful planning because of the different audiences and choosing appropriate styles for the various ways of disseminating. Let us now consider some ways to publish research. Below is guidance for writing an executive summary for publication in newsletters or websites.

Executive summary

The executive summary may consist of about four (A4) pages. It provides an overview and summary of the whole content and guides the reader through the various sections of the report.

Introduction

This needs to tell the reader about the background to the research and its context. Why was it undertaken? It may be that it initiated a new policy, or addressed an issue in an institutional development plan. It is possible it was commissioned by policy makers. Details of any published literature or documents which set the scene must be included.

Aims

Aims and objectives must be stated clearly; what the researcher was hoping to find out or achieve.

Review of relevant literature

The length of this section and what is included here needs to be decided on in relation to the total length and the audience. It would be useful to include a list of the recent and relevant documents and readings consulted when the action research was carried out.

Planned activities

A list of activities planned for the project should be provided. This section will be very useful and of significant interest to other practitioners who may wish to replicate the project in full or parts of it. The sources of any published materials used must be included. Details of what may have been designed for the project and the rationale for using these materials would be useful too.

Mode of enquiry

The mode of enquiry would be action research in the context of this report. Details of what sources of data were used and how the ethical issues were addressed (see Chapter 5) should go in here. Brief details of how the data were analysed should also be included.

Findings

The main findings should be listed and supported by evidence. Tables and figures are fine to include, but extracts from interviews, field logs, quotes from colleagues, and documentary evidence such as examples of work and photographs will make the report interesting and more accessible for prac-titioners who will constitute the main audience.

Discussion

Here the findings are discussed in the light of other research and unexpected results are explained. Limitations of the findings are provided.

Conclusions

These should be stated relating to the aims.

Implications for practice and policy

These require a comment on the implications for other practitioners. If researching a policy issue, the report will be of interest and significance to policy makers. Making recommendations for both practitioners and policy makers as appropriate may also be relevant.

Newsletters or webpages

Newsletters may be in a written format, if they are to be distributed to a local area. These could also be placed on the website of an institution which is then accessible to large audiences through search engines sharing the research globally. In all cases, it is important for researchers to have the audience in mind. For example, a newsletter for patients needs to be very focused and relatively short, providing a summary of what was done and what the outcomes were. On the other hand, a newsletter for professional colleagues – in print or on the website – can be longer, as the audience would want to know more details about the project and where they can get more information if they wish. The need for clarity and a visually pleasing presentation cannot be over emphasized. Below is an example of a short report published on the webpage of a research and development centre at an academic institution. The project aimed to work out how to introduce methods for assessing the quality of care in general practices.

Example of a Short Report
Public release of information: a developmental evaluation (pride) (Marshall et al.) at National Primary Care Research and Development Centre
http://www.npcrdc.ac.uk/projectdetail.cfm?id=104

This project used an action research approach and was carried out between September 2002 and August 2005. It was initiated and coordinated by researchers from the universities of Manchester and Swansea. Key participants in the project were members of the public in four localities in England and Wales, working in partnership with the staff in their general practices and NHS managers. They found that:

- the public regarded the current sources of information about general practice as inadequate and wanted to be better informed;
- the public were more interested in information about the context and availability of services than about the performance of individual practices;
- the public do not like performance league tables and most did not want to use comparative information to choose between practices, preferring to work in partnership with their existing practice to improve services;
- the public wished to be clear about the source of information so they could make personal judgements about its trustworthiness.

These findings were developed with the help of cognitive science that provided guidance about how to communicate with non-expert audiences and were used to create hard-copy guides and a website. In their design, content, and presentation format, these sources provided the most sophisticated examples until then, of how to produce information about general practices which was accessible and useful to the public. As a result of this project the authors recommended that future policy and practice in the area of producing health information sources needed to:

(Continued)

(Continued)

- build on the good will and sense of responsibility that the public has for their local practices and not treat primary healthcare in the UK as a consumer product;
- engage the public by building incrementally on the relatively modest kinds of information that they said they wanted at this time, rather than alienating them with too much or too sophisticated data;
- accept that the presentational format of information sources is as important as the content;
- encourage local communities to work with their local practices and NHS managers on the development of information sources;
- undertake further research into the information needs of minority groups, the factors influencing the public's demand for information, and the relative importance and interaction between 'hard' performance data and patients' personal experiences.

The *Pride Handbook* was designed to help people to develop local reports describing the range and quality of services on offer from general practices. It was written for patients and members of the public who used general practice. The website continues to be developed and is being rolled out to a large sample of practices in England and Wales.

Who will be the audience?

First researchers need to consider who the audience will be. If this will be international, researchers need to be careful about the terminology and language they use. The context of the work must be clear. Avoiding acronyms and abbreviations used in one country, which may not be understood by an international readership, is useful here.

Publishing in professional journals

By writing in a professional journal researchers will be sharing their research – both the research process and findings – with healthcare professionals. They would be using the sort of information as was used in the report, but would need to use a different style to engage with the reader. Again, sharing the sources of the materials and resources used or designed, with examples, is helpful because busy practitioners will appreciate having access to tried and tested materials. Using case study examples and anecdotes can make the story more powerful and reader-friendly. When researchers share their experiences as action researchers they must not forget to include any problems they may have encountered, which then adds to the realism of carrying out research as part of our professional work. Unanticipated problems and barriers to progress are common within the realities of healthcare settings and institutions. Writing collaboratively or with a 'writing mate' can make the process of writing less stressful. Looking out for specialized journals arising from specific professional associations (e.g. the *Nursing Standard* which is published by the Royal College of Nursing) is worthwhile because they might be more willing to publish clinically-oriented articles. It may also be helpful to researchers to write a summary of the research and to send this to the editor of a journal asking whether they would be interested in considering the article for publication. In our experience journal editors of professional journals are very keen to publish work from practitioners who constitute their main readership. Practitioners who work with us at the university often say that they see the experience of writing papers for professional journals as a useful first step towards writing papers for academic journals. There are a number of journals which publish action research. Their editors would obviously be very keen to publish good quality projects.

Publishing in academic outlets

It may be that an action researcher has decided to present the research at a research conference or write a paper for an academic journal. Here are some useful points to achieving this. If this is for an academic journal, then the following steps could be taken:

Preparation stage

- Looking at the websites of academic journals to see samples of journals and published papers. Most university libraries will subscribe to medical journals and students or those working with a member of the university staff should be able to look at these journals on-line.
- Academic journals that arise out of professional associations might be more receptive to action research, for example, the *International Journal of Mental Health Nursing* which is the official journal of the Australian College of Mental Health Nurses.
- Downloading abstracts and full copies of papers which are of interest.
- Making a note of what the journal is looking for. Reading the guidance notes in the journal which outline the aims of the journal, its audience, the format and style, and the suggested wordage is a good starting point.
- Selecting one or two of the most suitable journals to submit research output.

Writing an academic paper
The following guidance may be helpful:

- Choosing which journal to publish with, bearing in mind the reasons for publishing.

- Preparing an abstract. This is a short summary of what a paper is about. The author guidelines will show how it should be presented. Some journals will like a clear structure while others may not.
- Writing a draft paper using the format of the particular journal to be targetted while staying focused and articulating the theoretical stance. Showing research that others have completed in areas related to the research. Robust methodology and the collection and analysis of data are important aspects that reviewers will look for. Finally, it is most important to highlight what new knowledge the study has contributed to existing knowledge and its significance to healthcare.
- Completing the references and bibliography. Using an automated referencing tool such as 'Endnote' will make this task easier.
- Asking someone who has had experience of publishing to critique the article (preferably someone who has not been involved in the project) and to read it for clarity and language. Any links with the local university as part of the project may mean tutors would be prepared to read the draft and make comments.
- Revising the draft and sending the paper to the selected journal for consideration.
- In most cases, journal editors will ask for some revisions before publishing. A rejection letter may sometimes be sent out. Comments can be noted, the article can be re-presented and sent to another journal. More often than not, it will be published.

Options for presenting a study in academic journal

As with dissertations, there are options for the way an action research project might be presented in an article. The emphasis might be on:

- the research protocol;
- the process i.e. the phases of a project;
- the findings of the project;
- the recommendations for practice and policy.

Alternatively there may be a combination of two or more of the above.

Below is an exercise to test the reader's understanding of how articles might be presented, using abstracts of three articles that have been published in academic journals. Try to determine the differences in presentation between them.

Example 7.4   An action research protocol to strengthen system-wide inter-professional learning and practice (Braithwaite et al., 2007, available at BMC Health Services open access)

Abstract

Background

Inter-professional learning (IPL) and inter-professional practice (IPP) are thought to be critical determinants of effective care, improved quality and safety, and enhanced provider morale, yet few empirical studies have demonstrated this. Whole-of-system research is even less prevalent. We aim to provide a four year, multi-method, multi-collaborator action research programme of IPL and IPP in defined, bounded health and education systems located in the Australian Capital Territory (ACT). The project is funded by the Australian Research Council under its industry Linkage Programme.

Methods/Design

The programme of research will examine in four inter-related, prospective studies, progress with IPL and IPP across tertiary education providers, professional education, regulatory and registration bodies, the ACT health system's streams of care activities and teams, units and wards of the provider facilities of the ACT health system. One key focus will be on push-pull mechanisms, i.e., how the education sector creates student-enabled IPP and the health sector demands IPL-oriented practitioners. The studies will examine four research aims and meet 20 research project objectives in a comprehensive evaluation of ongoing progress with IPL and IPP.

Discussion

IPP and IPL are said to be the cornerstones of health system reforms. We will measure progress across an entire health system and the clinical and professional education systems that feed into it. The value of multi-methods, partnership research and a bi-directional push-pull model of IPL and IPP will be tested. Widespread dissemination of results to practitioners, policymakers, managers and researchers will be a key project goal.

Example 7.5   Social and structural violence and power relations in mitigating HIV risk of drug-using women in survival sex work (Shannon et al., 2008, *Social Science & Medicine*, 66: 911–921)

Abstract

High rates of violence among street-level sex workers have been described across the globe, while in cities across Canada the disappearance and victimization of drug-using women in survival sex work is ongoing. Given the pervasive levels of violence faced by sex workers over the last decades, and extensive harm reduction and HIV prevention efforts operating in Vancouver, Canada, this research aimed to explore the role of social and structural violence and power relations in shaping the HIV risk environment and prevention practices of women in survival sex work. Through a participatory-action research

(Continued)

(Continued)

project, a series of focus group discussions were conceptualized and co-facilitated by sex workers, community and research partners with a total of 46 women in early 2006. Based on thematic, content and theoretical analysis, the following key factors were seen to both directly and indirectly mediate women's agency and access to resources, and their ability to practice HIV prevention and harm reduction: at the micro-level, boyfriends as pimps and the 'everyday violence' of bad dates; at the meso-level, a lack of safe places to take dates, and the adverse impacts of local policing; and at the macro-level, dope-sickness and the need to sell sex for drugs. Analysis of the narratives and daily lived experiences of women sex workers highlights the urgent need for a renewed HIV prevention strategy that moves beyond a solely individual-level focus to structural and environmental interventions, including legal reforms, that facilitate 'enabling environments' for HIV prevention.

Example 7.6　The process of practice redesign in delirium care for hospitalised older people: a participatory action research study. (Day et al., 2009, *International Journal of Nursing Studies*, 46: 13–22)

Abstract

Background

In 2007 three researchers completed a six-month study in one 32-bed acute care medical ward in a large hospital in New South Wales, Australia. The problem drawn to the attention of researchers was that approximately 60% of older people were delirious on arrival or developed incident delirium during their hospital stay. A lack of recognition, underreporting and inadequate care responses to delirium in hospitalised older people signalled a major practice problem.

Aim

To collaboratively explore ways in which clinical practice could be improved.

Method

We selected Participatory Action Research (PAR) as the methodology to involve health practitioners in practice redesign. PAR is a process in which 'we', the researchers and participants, systematically work together in cycles of 'looking, thinking and acting'. Delirium and the high percentage of older people who succumb to this condition was the main practice problem requiring a response.

Eight volunteer clinicians and three researchers met weekly as a group for 13 sessions over six months. Clinicians set the agenda for the redesign of practice. Raising awareness about delirium and its prevention were the selected action strategies. A delirium alert protocol was developed for implementation by the clinicians and later evaluation as a separate study.

Findings

There was evidence that practice had changed. Physical and chemical restraints had not been used for three months subsequent to the study's completion. The nurse manager reported that early detection strategies had prevented episodes of acute hyperactive delirium. Whilst there continued to be older people admitted with a diagnosis of delirium, there were fewer incidences of delirium developing on the ward and there was less disruption to other patients, especially at night. The strategy of raising the awareness of delirium in older people was successful. We are confident that working collaboratively with practitioners is the way to bring evidence to practice in delirium care for older people in acute care settings.

On reading the three abstracts, it should become apparent that the first example was about a protocol for an action research project, the second abstract focused on the findings that the project reported, and the third contained a detailed discussion of the action research process. These are all perfectly acceptable publishing formats so long as the authors make it clear what they intend to write about near the beginning of the article.

A checklist for reviewing a paper before sending it for publication

We have often found the list of criteria used by research associations and journals to be very useful for reviewing papers before they are submitted. Rejections are part of the academic writing process, but we can enhance the quality of the paper by addressing the following questions:

- Has the background to the study been clearly stated and why the study was carried out?
- What type of study was it? In the context of this book, it would be using an action research approach. Why was this method of inquiry selected?
- What were the aims or objectives?
- Has an analysis of the theory and research which informed the study been included?
- Has study design been articulated carefully?
- Are the methods of data collection and analysis clear?
- Has the study addressed any ethical issues?
- Have the limitations of the study been included?

- What contribution has the study made to the existing knowledge base?
- Are there any special aspects to carrying out the action research which the reader may find useful, in terms of personal learning or the process itself?

Summary

This chapter dealt with report writing which can often be the final stage for the action researcher. After the choice of topic, cycles of enquiry, data collection and analysis, the end would be in sight. The report is the ultimate activity serving the purpose of portraying the action research as an attempt to investigate a phenomenon and disseminate the findings on which to base further practical changes. The target audience, their interests and dispositions need to be borne in mind. Although dissertations or theses will have to follow specified structures provided by institutions, a general set of guidelines for writing dissertations was provided. A collection of extracts from action research projects were given to help the reader relate to the style and content of a dissertation. One example of an abstract from a nursing doctorate student, who had carried out an institution-based study, was included. The possibility of disseminating action research findings as posters, presentations and via newsletters and web pages was also discussed. Guidance was provided on how to write professional and academic journal articles. Examples were given to help the reader understand the various formats required for publishing action research.

Further reading

McNiff, J. and Whitehead, J. (2005) *All You Need To Know About Action Research*. London: SAGE.

Stringer, E.T. and Genat, W.J. (2004) *Action Research in Health*. Upper Saddle River, NJ: Pearson Prentice-Hall.

Winter, R. and Munn-Giddings, C. (2001) *A Handbook for Action Research in Health and Social Care*. London: Routledge.

Glossary of key terms

If the reader feels mystified by some terms in the research language, here are some explanations. These are only meant as a starting point in order to explore them further as the reader proceeds with any research.

Action research is an approach employed by practitioners for improving practice as part of a process of change. The research is context-bound and participative.

Coding is a process used for data analysis. It involves assigning a code to help with the interpretation of segments of the data.

Data are the information researchers collect. They may generate a lot of it as tape-recorded interviews, questionnaires, field diaries, and documentary evidence. It is very important that researchers design an effective, personal system to organize the data.

Data analysis in general terms, is the process of making interpretations of the data collected and, possibly, of constructing theories based on interpretations.

Documentary analysis relates to the process of analysing and interpreting the data that are gathered via documents. For example, government documents, health policies, the minutes of meetings, diaries or health records are studied and analysed to make observations.

Emergent quality in action research means an investigator making adjustments to their plans in response to on-going assessments. The cyclic nature of action research allows them to take account of a quality which has emerged that was not exhibited in a previous cycle.

Epistemology is about theories of knowledge and about how we come to know these.

Ethics   is concerned with ethical principles and adherence to professional codes. These principles need to be at the centre of the whole research process.

Field notes and field diaries   are entries made by researchers based on their observations and thoughts. Field notes do not have to be in written form and audio tapes and video tapes can be employed to gather authentic data. In participant observations, the use of field notes can be particularly helpful.

Focus group interviews   are a commonly used data-gathering method, where a small group of people is interviewed together and led by a facilitator/moderator.

Objectivity   is a complex term, but in practice it involves the attempted avoidance of any intrusion of a researcher's preconceptions or value judgements. Objectivity is a means of avoiding bias and prejudice in interpretations.

Ontology   is the theory of being. It is the study of how things exist in the world, whether they exist subjectively or independent of the observer.

Participant observer   is used when researchers are involved in what is being studied. In action research we are likely to be involved in the project as participant observers.

Qualitative/quantitative methods   simply put, describe qualitative data as being in the form of descriptions using words whereas quantitative data will involve numbers. The debate as to which methods are more valid goes on; we recommend selecting methods which are likely to provide appropriate data for the purpose at hand.

Reflexivity   is the process by which researchers will reflect on their values, biases, personal background, and situations in shaping their interpretations.

Reliability   means we can describe a study as reliable if it can be replicated by another researcher.

Subjectivity   means the personal views and the commentaries of a researcher can sometimes be viewed as bias, but this does not have to be the case. If they declare the possible subjective nature of their statements or personal judgements and provide justifications for these then this can be powerful in constructing arguments within action research.

Triangulation a way of establishing the validity of findings. The researcher collects data from multiple sources involving multiple contexts, personnel, and methods. The process of triangulation involves sharing and checking the data with those involved. This should lead to researchers being able to construct a more reliable picture.

Validity of the data is achieved by sound and robust data collection, sharing all the data sources with participants, and a consensus on accurate interpretations. Different interpretations of a situation may add to a debate and lead to the personal and professional development of the researchers involved. The action research cycle is a validating process in itself.

Useful websites

www.uea.ac.uk/care/
Centre for Applied Research in Education (CARE) in the University of East Anglia, which provides guidance and links to other networks.

www.parnet.org/
Participatory Action Research Network, which offers useful resources and links.

www.bath.ac.uk/edsa/w/
Action Research at Bath University. See also
www.triangle.co.uk (*Action Research*, an academic journal which publishes studies of interest to action researchers).

http://arj.sagepub.com

www. scu.edu.au/schools/gcm/arhome.html
Action Research resources at Southern Cross University, Australia.

www.did.stu.mmu.ac.uk/carnnew/
The Collaborative Action Research Network provides details of research publications and research conferences.

www. sagepub.co.uk/
SAGE publishes a number of useful journals.

www.educ.queensu.ca/-ar
A university-based site.

www.nice.orh.uk
National Institute for Health and Clinical Excellence in the UK, for evidence and clinical guidance.

www.dh.gov.uk/policyandguidance/researchanddevelopment/fs/en
Provides health-related research and development activities in England.

www. invo.org.uk/
INVOLVE, a national advisory group funded by the UK government's Department of Health, aims to promote public involvement in the National Health Service.

www.dh.gov.uk/
Department of Health website which provides information on research and development and government-supported research programmes.

www.tandf.co.uk/journals/titles
Gives journal details of *Educational Action Research*.

References

Auerbach, C.F. and Silverstein, L.B. (2003) *Qualitative Data: An Introduction to Coding and Analysis*. New York: New York University Press.

Austin, W., Goble, E., Strang, V., Mitchell, A. et al. (2009) 'Supporting relationships between family and staff in continuing care settings', *Journal of Family Nursing*, 15 (3): 360–380.

Baron, S. (2009) 'Evaluating the patient journey approach to ensure health care is centred on patients', *Nursing Times*, 105: 22 (early online publication, last accessed July 2009).

Bazeley, P. (2007) *Qualitative Data Analysis with NVivo*. London: SAGE.

Beringer, A. and Julier, H. (2009) 'Time off the ward: an action research approach to reducing nursing time spent accompanying children to X-ray', *Paediatric Nursing*, 21(2): 33–35.

Blaikie, N. (1993) *Approaches to Social Inquiry*. London: Polity.

Blaxter, L., Hughes, C. and Tight, M. (1996) *How to Research*. Buckingham: Open University Press.

Bloor, M., Frankland, J., Thomas, M. and Robson, K. (2001) *Focus Groups in Social Research*. London: SAGE.

Braithwaite, J., Westbrook, J.I., Foxwell, A.R., Boyce, R., Devinney, T., Budge, M., Murphy, K., Ryall, M.A., Beutel, J., Vanderheide, R., Renton, E. Travaglia, J., Stone, J., Barnard, A., Greenfield, D., Corbett, A., Nugus, P. and Clay-Williams, R. (2007) 'An action research protocol to strengthen system-wide inter-professional learning and practice', *BMC Health Services Research,* Open Access.

Bridges, J., Fitzgerald, L. and Meyer, J. (2007) 'New workforce roles in healthcare: exploring the longer-term journal of organizational innovations', *Journal of Health Organization and Management*, 21 (4/5): 381–392.

Buckland, S., Hayes, H., Ostrer, C., Royle, J. and Tarpey, M. et al. (2007) *Public Information Pack (PIP): How to Get Actively Involved in NHS, Public Health and Social Care Research*. London: INVOLVE.

Burrell, G. and Morgan, G. (1979) *Sociological Paradigms and Organizational Analysis*. London: Heinemann.

Carr, W. and Kemmis, S. (1986) *Becoming Critical: Education, Knowledge and Action Research*. London: Falmer.

Checkland, P. and Scholes, J. (1999) *Soft Systems Methodology in Action*. Chichester: Wiley.

Cohen, L. and Manion, L. (1994) *Research Methods in Education*. London: Routledge.

Creswell, J.W. (2009) *Research Design: Qualitative, Quantitative, and Mixed Methods Approaches*. Thousand Oaks, CA: SAGE.

Dadds, M. and Hart, S. (2001) *Doing Practitioner Research Differently*. Sussex: Taylor and Francis.

Dahlgren, G. and Whitehead, W. (1993) 'Tackling inequalities in health: What can we learn from what has been tried?'. Working paper prepared for the Kings Fund International Seminar on Tackling Inequalities in Health. Ditchley Park, Oxfordshire, Kings Fund.

Day, J., Higgins, I. and Koth, T. (2009) 'The process of practice redesign in delirium care for hospitalized older people: a participatory action research study', *International Journal of Nursing Studies*, 46: 13–22.

Denzin, N.K. and Lincoln, Y.S. (1994) *Handbook of Qualitative Research*. Thousand Oaks, CA: SAGE.

Department of Health (2001) *Essence of Care*. London: DoH.

Dickinson, A., Welch, C., Ager, L. and Costar, A. (2005) 'Hospital mealtimes: action research for change?', *Proceedings of the Nutrition Society*, 64: 269–275.

Dolan, A.L., Koshy, E., Waker, M. and Goble, C.M. (2004) 'Access to bone densitometry increases general practitioners' prescribing for osteoporosis in steroid treated patients', *Ann. Rheum Dis*. 63(92) (Feb): 183–186.

Eden, C. and Huxham, C. (1996) 'Action research for the study of organizations', in S. Clegg and W. Nord (eds), *A Handbook of Organization Studies*. London and Thousand Oaks, CA: SAGE.

Elliot, J. (1991) *Action Research for Educational Change*. Buckingham: Open University Press.

Feldman, A. (2008) 'Does academic culture support translational research?', *CTS: Clinical and Translational Science*, 1(2): 87–88.

Fenton, W. (2008) 'Introducing a post-fall assessment algorithm into a community rehabilitation hospital for older adults', *Nursing Older People*, 20 (10): 36–39.

Fink, A. (2005) *Conducting Research Literature Reviews: From the Internet to Paper*. London: SAGE.

Fontana, A. and Fret, J. (2005) 'The interview from neutral stance to political involvement', in N. Denzin and Y. Lincoln (eds), *The SAGE Handbook of Qualitative Research*. Thousand Oaks, CA: SAGE.

Gall, M., Gall, J. and Borg, W. (2007) *Educational Research: An Introduction*. Upper Saddle River, NJ: Pearson International.

Gaskell, G. (2000) 'Individual and group interviewing', in M.W. Bauer and G. Gaskell (eds), *Qualitative Researching with Text, Image and Sound*. London: SAGE.

Glaser, B. and Strauss, A. (1967) *The Discovery of Grounded Theory*. Chicago, IL: Aldine.

Grant, A. and Robling, M. (2006) 'Introducing undergraduate medical teaching into general practice: an action research study', *Medical Teacher*, 28 (7): e192–e197.

Green, L.W. (2004/2006) 'If we want more evidence-based practice, we need more practice-based evidence'. Available at http://www.green.net (last accessed April 2006).

Greenwood, D. and Levin, M. (1998) *Introduction to Action Research*. Thousand Oaks, CA: SAGE.

Guba, E.G. and Lincoln, Y.S. (1990) 'The alternative paradigm dialog', in E.G. Guba (ed.), *The Paradigm Dialog*. Newbury Park, CA: SAGE.

Guba, E.G. and Lincoln, Y.S. (2005) 'Paradigmatic controversies and contradictions and emerging confluences', in N.K. Denzin and Y.S. Lincoln (eds), *The SAGE Handbook of Qualitative Research*. London: SAGE.

Habermas, J. (1971) *Towards a Rational Society*. London: Heinemann.

Habermas, J. (1984) *Towards a Theory of Communicative Action* (Vol.1). Boston, MA: Beacon.

Halker, P.H., van Gijn, J., Kappelle, I.J., Koudstaal, P.J. and Algra, A. (2006) 'Aspirin plus dipyridamole versus aspiring alone after cerebreal ischaemia of arterial origin (ESPRIT): randomised controlled trial', *Lancet*, 20 (9523): 1665–1673.

Hampshire, A., Blair. M., Crown, N., Avery, A. and Williams, I. (1999) 'Action research: a useful method of promoting change in primary care?' *Family Practice*, 16 (3): 305–311.

Hart, E. and Bond, M. (1995) *Action Research for Health and Social Care*. London: Open University Press.

Hassett, G., Hart, D.J., Manek, N.J., Doyle, D.V. and Spector, T.D. (2003) 'Risk factors for progression of lumbar spine disc degeneration: the Chingford study', *Arthritis Rheum*, 48 (11) (Nov): 3112–3117.

Heron, J.(1996) *Co-operative Enquiry: Research into the Human Condition*. London: SAGE.

Hills, M., Mullet, J. and Carroll, S. (2007) 'Community-based participatory action research – transforming multidisciplinary practice in primary health care', *Rev. Panam Salud Publica, AM/J Public Health*, 21 (2/3): 125–35.

Holter, L. and Schwartz-Barcott, D. (1993) 'Action research – what is it? How has it been used? And how can it be used in nursing?' *Journal of Advanced Nursing*, 18: 298–304.

Hopkins, D. (2002) *A Teacher's Guide to Classroom Research*. Buckingham: Open University Press.

Hughes, I. (2008) 'Action research in healthcare', in P. Reason and H. Bradbury (eds), *The SAGE Handbook of Action Research: Participative Inquiry and Practice*. London: SAGE.

Isles, V. and Sutherland, K. (2001) '*Managing change in the NHS: organizational change: a review for healthcare managers, professionals and researchers*'. Report for the National Co-ordinating Centre for NHS Service Delivery and Organization R&D. London: London School of Hygiene and Tropical Medicine.

Jinks, C., Nio Ong, B. and O'Niell, T. (2009) 'The Keele community knee pain forum: action research to engage with stakeholders about the prevention of knee pain and disability', *Musculoskeletal Disorders. Bio Med Central*. Available at http://www.biomedcentral.com/1471-2474/10/85

Kelle, U. (2000) 'Computer-assisted analysis: coding and indexing', in M.W. Bauer and G. Gaskell (eds), *Qualitative Researching with Text, Image and Sound*. London: SAGE.

Kelly, D., Simpson, S. and Brown, P. (2002) 'An action research project to evaluate the clinical practice facilitator role for junior nurses in an acute hospital setting', *Journal of Clinical Nursing*, 11: 90–98.

Kemmis, K. and McTaggart, R. (1998) *An Action Research Planner*. Victoria: Deakin University.

Kemmis, K. and McTaggart, R. (2000) 'Participatory action research', in N. Denzin and Y. Lincoln (eds), *Handbook of Qualitative Research*. Thousand Oaks, CA: SAGE.

Koshy, E. (2008) 'The "Quality and Outcomes Framework": Improving care, but are all patients benefiting?', *JR Soc Med* 101 (9) (Sept): 432–433.

Koshy, E., Car, J. and Majeed, A. (2008) 'Effectiveness of mobile phone short message service (SMS) reminders for Ophthalmology outpatient appointments: an observational study'. Available at http://www.biomedcentral.com/1471-2415/8/9

Koshy, V. (2010) *Action Research for Improving Educational practice: A Step-by-Step Guide*. London: SAGE.

Kreuger, R.A. (1994) *Focus Groups: A Practical Guide for Applied Research*. Thousand Oaks, CA: SAGE.

Kumar, S., Little, P. and Britten, N. (2009) 'Why do general practitioners prescribe antibiotics for sore throats? Grounded theory interview study', *British Medical Journal*, 339: b4817.

Kvale, S. and Brinkman, S. (2009) *Interviews: Learning the Craft of Qualitative Research Interviewing*. London: SAGE.

Lakeman, R. and Glasgow, C. (2009) 'Introducing peer-group clinical supervision: An action research project', *International Journal of Mental Health Nursing*, 18: 204–210.

Leighton, K. (2005) 'Action research: the revision of services at one mental health rehabilitation unit in the north of England', *Journal of Psychiatric and Mental Health Nursing*, 12: 372–379.

Levin, M. and Greenwood, D. (2001) 'Pragmatic action research and the struggle to transform', in P. Reason and H. Bradbury (eds), *Handbook of Action Research: Participative Enquiry and Practice*. London: SAGE.

Lewin, K. (1946) 'Action research and minority problems', *Journal of Social Issues*, 2: 34–46.

Lincoln, Y. (2001) 'Engaging sympathies: relationship between action research and social constructivism', in P. Reason and H. Bradbury (eds), *Handbook of Action Research: Participative Enquiry and Practice*. London: SAGE.

Lindsey, E. and McGuinness, L. (1998) 'Significant elements of community involvement in participatory action research: evidence from a community project', *Journal of Advanced Nursing*, 28 (5): 1106–1114.

Lingard, L., Albert, M. and Levinson, W. (2008) 'Grounded theory, mixed methods, and action research', *British Medical Journal*, 337: 459–461.

Locke, L., Spirduso, W. and Silverman, S. (2007) *Proposals that Work: A Guide for Planning Dissertations and Grant Proposals*. Thousand Oaks, CA: SAGE.

Marincowitz, G. (2003) 'How to use participatory action research in primary care', *Family Practice*, 20: 595–600.

Marshall, M., Noble, J., Davies, H., Waterman, H., Walshe, K., Sheaff, R. and Elwyn, G. (2006) 'Development of an information source for patients and the public about general practice services: an action research study', *Health Expectations* 9: 265–274 (University of Manchester).

Mason, J. (2002) *Researching Your Own Practice: The Discipline of Noticing*. London: RoutledgeFalmer.

McKeller, L., Pincombe, J. and Henderson, A. (2009) 'Encountering the culture of midwifery practice on the postnatal ward during action research: an impediment to change', *Women and Birth* (doi:10.1016/j.wombi.2009.02.003).

Mertler, C. (2006) *Action Research: Teachers as Researchers in the Classroom*. Thousand Oaks, CA: SAGE.

Meyer, J. (1995) 'Stages in the process: a personal account', *Nurse Researcher*, 2: 24–37.

Meyer, J. (2000) 'Using qualitative methods in health related action research', *British Medical Journal*, 320: 178–181.

Meyer, J. (2006) 'Action research', in K. Gerrish and A. Lacey (eds), *The Research Process in Nursing*. Oxford: Blackwell.

Miles, M. and Huberman, M. (1994) *Qualitative Data Analysis*. Beverly Hills, CA: SAGE.

Mitchell, A., Conlon, A., Armstrong, M. and Ryan, A. (2005) 'Towards rehabilitative handling in caring for patients following stroke: a participatory action research project', *International Journal for Older People Nursing*, 14 (3a): 3–12.

Morrison, B. and Lilford, R. (2001) 'How can action research apply to health services?', *Qualitative Health Research*, 11 (4): 436–449.

Munday, J. (2006) 'Identity in focus: the use of focus groups to study the collective identity', *Sociology*, 40 (91): 89–105.

National Health Service (NHS) (2005) *A Short Guide to NHS Foundation Trusts* (Gateway 5531). London: DoH.

NRES (2009) 'Public involvement in research'. Available at http://nres.npsa.uk/patients-and-the public-involvement-in-research (last accessed 29 July 2009).

O'Dochartaigh, N. (2007) *Internet Research Skills*. London: SAGE.

O'Leary, Z. (2004) *The Essential Guide to Doing Research*. London: SAGE.

Oliver, D., Hopper, A. and Seed, P. (2000) 'Do hospital fall prevention programs work? A systematic review', *Journal of the American Geriatrics Society*, 48(12):1679–1689.

Parkin, P. (2009) *Managing Change in Healthcare: Using Action Research*. London: SAGE

Punch, K.F. (2009) *Introduction to Research Methods in Education*. London: SAGE.

Power, Z., Campbell, M., Kilcoyne, P., Kitchener, H. and Waterman, H. (2010) 'The Hyperemesis Impact of Symptoms Questionnaire', *International Journal of Nursing Studies*, 47: 67–77.

Reason, P. and Bradbury, H. (2001) *The SAGE Handbook of Action Research*, 1st edn. London: SAGE.

Reason, P. and Bradbury, H. (2006) *The SAGE Handbook of Action Research*, 2nd edn. London: SAGE.

Reason, P. and Bradbury, H. (2008) *The SAGE Handbook of Action Research*, 3rd edn. London: SAGE.

Reason, P. and Marshall, J. (2001) 'On working with graduate research students', in P. Reason and H. Bradbury (eds), *Handbook of Action Research: Participative Enquiry and Practice*. London: SAGE.

Reed, J. (2005) 'Using action research in nursing practice with older people: democratizing knowledge', *Journal of Clinical Nursing*, 14: 594–600.

Robson, C. (2002) *Real World Research*. Oxford: Blackwell.

Rossman, G. and Rallis, S. (1998) *Learning in the Field: An Introduction to Qualitative Research*. Thousand Oaks, CA: SAGE.

Royal College of Nursing (2007) *RCN Ethics Guidance for Nurses* (Revised Edition). London: RCN (www.rcn.org.uk, last accessed December 2008).

Ryan, R. and Happell, B. (2009) 'Learning from experience: Using action research to discover consumer needs in post seclusion debriefing', *International Journal of Mental Health*, 18: 100–107.

Schön, D. (1983) *The Reflective Practitioner*. New York: Basic.

Schön, D. (1991) *The Reflective Practitioner*. New York: Basic.

Shannon, K., Kerr, T., Allinott, S., Chettiar, J., Shoveller, J. and Tyndall, M.W. (2008) 'Social and structural violence and power relations in mitigating HIV risk of drug-using women in survival sex work', *Social Science & Medicine*, 66(4): 911–21.

Stenhouse, L. (1975) *An Introduction to Curriculum Research and Development*. London: Heinemann.

Stenhouse, L. (1983) *Authority, Education and Emancipation*. London: Heinemann.

Strauss, A. and Corbin, J. (1998) *Basic Qualitative Research*. London: SAGE.

Stringer, E. (1999) *Action Research*, 1st edn. Thousand Oaks, CA: SAGE.

Stringer, E. (2004) *Action Research*, 2nd edn. Upper Saddle River, NJ: Pearson.

Stringer, E. (2007) *Action Research*. Thousand Oaks, CA: SAGE.

Stringer, E.T. and Genat, W.J. (2004) *Action Research in Health*. Upper Saddle River, NJ: Pearson Prentice-Hall.

Stringer, E., Guhathakurta, M. and Waddell, S. (2008) 'Guest editors' commentary action research and development', *Action Research*, 6 (2): 123–127.

Toulmin, S. and Gustavsen, B. (eds) (1996) *Beyond Theory: Changing Organizations through Participation*. Amsterdam: John Benjamins.

Van Deventer, C. and Hugo, J. (2005) 'Participatory action research in the teaching of primary healthcare nurses in Venda', *South African Family Practice*, 47 (2): 57–60.

Waterman, H. (1996) 'A comparison of action research with quality assurance?' *Nurse Researcher*, 3 (3): 15–23.

Waterman, H., Harker, R., MacDonald, H. and Waterman, C. (2005) 'Evaluation of an action research project in ophthalmic practice', *Journal of Advanced Nursing*, 52 (4): 389–398.

Waterman, H., Tillen, D., Dickson, R. and de Koning, K. (2001) 'Action research: a systematic review and guidance for assessment', *Health Technology Assessment*, 5 (23).

Webber, R. (1990) *Basic Content Analysis*. Thousand Oaks, CA: SAGE.

Welsh Assembly (2007) *Action Research Resource Pack*. Available at www.wales.gov.uk/cmoresearch

White, J. and Kudless, M. (2008) 'Valuing Autonomy, struggling for an identity and a collective voice, and seeking role recognition: community mental health nurses' perceptions of their roles', *Issues in Mental Health Nursing*, 29: 1066–1087.

Whitehead, D., Taket, A. and Smith, P. (2003) 'Action research in health promotion', *Health Education Journal*, 62(5).

Whitelaw, S., Beattie, A., Balogh, R. and Watson, J. (2003) *A Review of the Nature of Action Research*. Cardiff: Welsh Assembly Government.

Winter, R. (1996) 'Some principles and procedures for the conduct of action research', in O. Zuber-Skerritt (ed.), *New Directions in Action Research*. London: Falmer.

Winter, R. and Munn-Giddings, C. (2001) *A Handbook for Action Research in Health and Social Care*. London: Routledge.

Williams, A. (2009) 'Making diabetes education accessible for people with visual impairment', *The Diabetes Educator*, 35 (4): 612–621.

World Health Organization (1946) 'Preamble to the Constitution of the World Health Organization as adopted by the International Health Conference, New York, 19–22 June 1946', *Official Records of the World Health Organization*, 2(100).

Zuber-Skerritt, O. (ed.) (1996) *New Directions in Action Research*. London: Falmer.

Index

NOTE: Page numbers in *italic type* refer to figures and tables.